KNOCK K
TI

C000067810

To Proof-reader
Patsy,
Thanks a million
Barbara

By Barbara Goulden

'One million people commit suicide every year'
The World Health Organization

Knock Knock, Who's There?

Published by
Chipmunkapublishing
PO Box 6872
Brentwood
Essex CM13 1ZT
United Kingdom

http://www.chipmunkapublishing.com

Copyright © Barbara Goulden 2008

Edited by Mary Dow
Front Cover Design by Mark Sargent

Barbara Goulden

**For my sister and her friends,
who inspired this book.**

Chapter 1

SLUGS had slithered in through the cat flap overnight. Jane screwed up her face and suppressed a scream. She knew it was the rain and the largely uneaten bowl of cat food that had drawn the slugs in. One fat specimen lay bloated, presumably dead, in the middle of the dish. The cat would have to go.

But first she'd have to find some way of dealing with these stomach-churning, slimy aliens who had invaded her living space. No. She was ill. It wasn't her job. It wasn't even her damn cat. Beloved Sandy had forced the thing on her.

"It will be company in the new flat," her sister asserted.

And Sandy – Sandra really - always got her own way. Always knew what was best.

Tenants in these flats weren't even supposed to have pets. But Sandy wheedled and persisted, before finally turning up on the doorstep with the sharp-clawed kitten saying: "Jane you need something to love, something to be responsible for. This is the start of a new life for you, a chance to be part of a real community…"

Ha! The thing had its cute moments all right but it was forever crying for attention. If it went out Jane was worried it would go on the road. If it stayed in she didn't know how to entertain it. And fussy…God, if it didn't get the best quality cat food it just turned and stared at her before arching its back and heading for the door.

Knock Knock, Who's There?

Or rather the newly acquired cat flap, paid for by high-flying, fast-talking Sandy and her pony-tailed new partner Roger.

"It'll be more convenient for you," they said, before jetting off for a skiing holiday in the Pyrenees.

Jane's next door neighbour, who she tried to have as little to do with as possible, had already christened the cat 'Mr C' and was forever trying to lure it into her own, more comfortable flat, with tins of sardines. No wonder it wouldn't eat cut-price Kat Munchies. Only the slugs fancied them.

After several attempts to lift the dead, bloated one out of the food bowl by balancing it on the tip of her umbrella, Jane gave up. She sat down, smoked her last two cigarettes, and howled.

*****

In the end it was George, the manic depressive from upstairs who disposed of the slugs.

Fortunately, George was on an upswing and full of enthusiasm for all creatures great and gross.

Tactfully, he told Jane: "I was having a lie down and could hear you was a bit upset."

Jane didn't bother to tell him how much more upset she got at four o'clock in the morning when he was playing all his old Pink Floyd and Jimi Hendrix records at full blast.

She'd been trying to shape her thick, dark hair with the kitchen scissors. It hadn't been an entirely successful trim. She'd only got one of her long-dangling earrings back in when the kitten growled and pounced on the other lying on the sofa.

"D'you fancy going bowling?" said George, tattooed and rippling with muscles.

"No. But thanks," said Jane, her eyes resting anxiously on the plastic supermarket bag he'd used for the slug removal job. She imagined it writhing. The cat tensed over the earring, waiting for it to move.

"You don't want him as a reward, do you?" asked Jane, nodding towards Mr so-called C.

George was shocked. "You've only had the thing five minutes – give it a chance! Anyway, it'd bring on my asthma. Got to go. See you later."

Not if I see you first, thought Jane, picking up the phone to ring her mother. She didn't know why but a good rant at her mother often made Jane feel better. After all, it was her dear mother's fault that she was in this God-forsaken flat with loonies for neighbours.

She'd hardly started jabbing in the numbers when Wendy, the warden – "I'm not really a warden, I'm just here to lend a hand in times of trouble" - came knocking on the door.

"Bit of a problem Jane? Are you all right?"

The faithless kitten immediately began purring round Wendy's legs.

"Oh hello, Mr C, you haven't been round for your elevenses this morning," simpered the warden.

"Elevenses!" Jane could have spit. No wonder the cat was bursting at the seams and she had slugs.

"No. No problem. Except that I'm out of cigarettes. Perhaps you can pop back later?"

"Oh! Well yes, of course," sniffed Wendy.

Knock Knock, Who's There?

Jane was still closing the door on the warden when she remembered to trap traitorous Mr so-called C in her poky little bathroom. No doubt it would pee on the floor. She didn't want to go out but anything was better than another lecture from bloody Wendy.

One thing she and all the other six tenants of Peacehaven Mansions knew, without ever discussing it, was that you never consort with The Enemy. Those on the other side. The ones with the power to lock you up and throw away the key.

Not that being looked after didn't have its attractions, Jane thought as she marched up the busy road. On bad days she found herself looking back almost with nostalgia to the times when nurses made all her decisions, cooked her dinner and were responsible for getting her up in the mornings. It was only the other things they could also do under the all-embracing Mental Health Act.

All the tenants of the house had been in hospital with some form of psychiatric condition. Jane happened to know the doctors had misdiagnosed her case. But as a frequent hospital "service user" she'd still been offered her own flat carved out of this rather grand Victorian monstrosity that had evidently seen better days.

Bit like us, mused Jane, who 27 years earlier had begun a university degree with three good A levels and enough confidence to take on the world. Now her concentration was completely up the spout. If she picked up a decent Agatha Christie in a charity shop she could never remember whodunit even though she'd read every single one of the books before.

Peacehaven Mansions was meant to be another prime example of care in the community. Nobody mentioned the fact that this particular community cared so much they'd held at least four protest meetings before Jane and the others had even moved in.

*****

It was at the end of the first year of her sociology degree that Jane dropped out. Since then she'd been in and out of hospital more times than she cared to remember and twice held under section for her own safety. There'd only ever been one course of ECT – electro-convulsive therapy – but that was enough. Even the doctors didn't know how strapping you down and administering 240 volts of electricity was supposed to unscramble the brain.

They only knew it worked. Sometimes.

Shock treatment was the one memory that remained crystal clear in Jane's jumbled mind. And the fear of it ever happening again would never go away.

Of course, these days nobody would admit her condition was actually physical rather than mental. In compensation-obsessed Britain, Jane understood all too well that no doctor was going to admit past mistakes. Instead she had evolved her own home-brewed philosophy for survival on the 'outside'. You had to be cheerful with the community psychiatric nurses, in case you looked depressed, pretend to be interested in their personal lives and tinpot alternative health remedies, and turn up on a regular basis to have major tranquilisers pumped into your bottom. Oh yes, and never, ever admit to hearing voices.

Not that Jane's voices had ever stopped.

*****

It was cold on the way to the newsagents and Jane had been in too much of a hurry to grab a coat or comb her hair after its haphazard trim. Her clothes came mainly from supermarkets and second-hand shops, which were her favourite sources of cut-price fashion. She had a good eye for colour but couldn't stand anything tight on her body which meant her tops were always too baggy and hip-fitting skirts way too long.

She was still wearing the single earring – one of her more flamboyant favourites with an iridescent crescent moon above showers of stars.

Jane always noticed people on the road giving her funny, sideways glances. Of course, everyone knew about the inmates of the double-fronted Peacehaven Mansions. Or Fruitcake Towers, as some wag had dubbed it.

The name had apparently stuck. It had been used one day when Jane was waiting in a queue at the post office. Everyone laughed, then somebody noticed her, and the line went quiet. There was a shuffling of feet, a clearing of throats. Most people looked the other way. Except for one oblivious old codger in a herringbone overcoat who had gone on and on about the house in its glory days when it had landscaped grounds and a full set of servants. He was furious about the unsightly fire escape the council had insisted was bolted to the top floor and seemed to know all about the row of old service bells on the wall of the central stairwell. Jane's flat had its own side entrance so she didn't pass that way very often. But joker Winston, music-lover George and agoraphobic Renee, who lived upstairs, were always pretending they could ring down to Wendy for a tea tray.

Listening to the old man Jane thought if this was the worst the neighbours could do - reminisce about the house before it had dry rot – then she could cope.

But it hadn't been the worst.

Within the first week of moving in, Ray, the anorexic chef who lived at the back of the house, had been humiliated in the local pub and ended up spilling his pint down his trousers.

He told Jane how a gang of middle-aged bruisers were glaring at him for most of the night until one balding lout had walked right up and just told him to 'bugger off.'

"We don't want your sort in the Queen's 'Ed," another yob had shouted. "And you can tell all your mates at the loony home they won't be welcome here either…"

The landlord had tried to defuse the situation and made some excuse about them all being drunk.

Knock Knock, Who's There?

One wavy-haired customer with a nose stud had bravely stood up and offered to have a game of darts with Ray. But when the thugs showed no sign of backing down the barman had politely asked Ray if he wouldn't be more 'comfortable' sitting in the lounge bar.

"I told him," said Ray, "I'd be more comfortable in a snake-pit but I still intend making this pub my local."

Jane had grinned at this part of the story. But poor, proud Ray - who'd once been the sous chef at a four star hotel in Birmingham - still came off worse. When he'd gone back the next night things had got even uglier with taunts like 'child molester' and "fucking-psycho" thrown about.

Despite continuing treatment, Ray never managed to eat very much and weighed a lot less than Jane. Beer was one of the very few tastes he'd managed to win back. He was so thin that glorious, drunken oblivion came quickly; though he still carried on drinking.

"I'm going back there tomorrow," he'd told Jane, who'd just filled the communal washing machine and offered to throw in his beer-soaked trousers.

Ray had been one of the first to take up residence in Peacehaven Mansions and his windows still had some of the original stained glass. They looked out on the overgrown remains of what must once have been landscaped grounds. When he wasn't in the pub Ray tended to keep himself to himself with the curtains closed. After Jane arrived he offered to swap flats because her place looked out onto a brick wall.

Barbara Goulden

Jane had said no; the brick wall was fine.

Chapter 2

It was on the way to the Pyrenees, driving between fields of sunflowers and sweetcorn that the future began to take on a golden glow for Sandy. It was Roger's turn to take the wheel of the hired Mondeo and they were singing together as they drove towards the French town of Pau on a glitteringly hot afternoon.

Contrary to Jane's assumption that the lovers had gone skiing, it was June and the snow was confined to the mountain peaks soaring above Pau.

They were an attractive, unlikely couple, though neither of them was young. Company director Sandy was a widow and lone parent. Roger was a divorcee who had given up a secure teaching job to play guitar in a series of professional and semi-professional rock and jazz bands.

"Money's not everything," he'd explained. "This is something I should have done years ago – now I'm living the dream before it's too late."

In the car he'd been secretly impressed by Sandy's ability to hold a tune. She'd kept quiet about her membership of a local choral society.

The holiday was the first time they had been alone together for any sustained length of time. Both knew the trip would lay bare exactly where their slow-burning, nearly 12-months-long relationship was going. And so far everything was going better than either of them could have hoped.

Except for Sandy's ankles that had started to swell in strappy new sandals too stylish to be comfortable. She hoped Roger hadn't noticed. Between mad bursts of song, she kept reminding him to slow down as they raced past ominous public notices informing motorists of how many accidents there'd been on each particular stretch of road over the past three years.

The French authorities were nothing if not thorough. As well as telling drivers there had been 25 deaths in five years on the N134 heading south, they'd erected faceless black metal figures on the actual spots where the tragedies occurred. Occasionally, there had been a smaller, child-sized figure that caused Sandy to stop singing and think about her daughter, Bella.

But only for a moment. Nothing could really dim her spirits as they finally reached the busy town. It took ages to find a parking spot. Sandy's feet were throbbing when they finally sank down to eat dinner in an old square, under a canopy of pale green leaves.

The food was fantastic. She'd restricted herself to just one small glass of red wine with her boeuf bourgignon followed by a sumptuous floating islands dessert. Roger had talked with some passion about his hopes for the future as a professional musician.

As he slowly polished off the rest of the bottle of red, then had a beer, he explained: "It's not that I want to be famous – I wrote what turned out to be a one hit wonder at the end of the 1980s. But I'm too old for that throwaway stuff now. I just want to be respected in the industry – brought in to do more gigs and session work – a lot more arrangements and composing. It's why I gave up the day job. Music's just too important."

The plan was to have an after-dinner stroll then drive straight on to their hotel, a further 20 kilometres up into the mountains. But on the walk back to the car they'd stumbled across a Ugandan band in the middle of a free performance in the main park. Within minutes they were dancing alongside an enthusiastic crowd of several hundred other holidaymakers. The place was still heaving at 11pm when the concert finished and everyone began streaming back to their hotels and favourite bars.

Roger insisted on congratulating each member of the band personally and ended up spending ages in animated – and complicated - conversation with a drummer who spoke little English. Sandy studied the illuminated trees, entranced by the range of colours. She watched as one leaf, which had yellowed early, spiralled to the ground at her feet. She picked it up as a keepsake, suddenly realising that the heat of the day was gone, her shoes were pinching like mad, and she was shivering. Roger handed her his jacket.

"What a fantastic night! Here, you need warming up, I'm way too caned to feel the cold. Still okay to drive? Or shall we book into a hotel here?"

"I'll be fine, once I'm back in the car," smiled Sandy, pressing close enough to pick up some of his body heat and standing on tip-toe to kiss his cheek.

"It was a wonderful evening. And the hotel knew we'd be late so they'll keep the room."

Once they were back in the car she swapped her sandals and adjusted the driver's seat.

"Perhaps we could come back here tomorrow night," she said, switching on the engine and laughing at Roger's glassy "lights-on-but-nobody-at-home" eyes. Even though she was still cold, she took off his jacket and flung it over him.

"Mmmm…there's some Chilean pipers on," said Roger, settling into a cocoon as warm air finally began to seep up and take the chill off the Mondeo.

"Brilliant musicians tonight. Really not up to driving. You okay?"

"I'm fine," Sandy assured him. "You have a nap - think I'll just give Mum a quick ring and check up on Bella."

She checked her watch, it was an hour earlier in England so her mother should be still up.

To her surprise it was 12-year-old Bella herself, who answered the phone.

"'Lo Mum, you having a good time?"

"Wonderful, but shouldn't you be in bed? It's school tomorrow."

"I've just finished a monster essay and was unwinding with a bit of *Sex In The City.*"

Sandy smiled. "You're trying to wind me up. Your gran wouldn't let you watch that – she wouldn't even approve of me watching it!"

"I know, it was worth a try though."

Knock Knock, Who's There?

"It's freezing here so I'm just trying to get warm. We've been watching a band in the park and it got really cold...."

Roger muttered from beneath his coat, then began to snore, softly.

"Roger sends his love, and remember we'll be back next Saturday, probably fairly early if we can get an overnight crossing."

"Great. Aunty Jane says she'll take me to the cinema tomorrow to see a remake of some old film she's keen on. Grandma says I'm not to bank on it but I reckon she'll turn up and take me – at least she won't be able to smoke when we're in there."

"No, but she'll probably keep nipping out at exciting moments and disturbing everyone else! Just make sure she sits in an aisle seat. Anyway, you're okay? Good. Put Grandma on and 'Go To Bed'. Night, night."

When Mary, Sandy's mother, came to the phone she said: "I knew you'd catch me out letting her stay up so late. But Bella deserved a little relaxation after working so hard. And don't forget I got both you and your sister to university!"

Even though one of us only graduated to a psychiatric ward, thought Sandy sadly.

Aloud, she said: "Yes mother, I'd just prefer it if Bella was relaxing in bed and not in front of the telly. Anyway, how're you holding up having practically a teenager living in the house all over again?"

"I rather like it. We're having fun. Well, I suppose I'm having fun but I think Bella's enjoying the change of scene..."

Mary lowered her voice: "I suspect she's going to start missing you over the weekend."

Sandy knew her mum was trying to make her feel wanted. After once more going over their estimated times of return, she felt reassured that all was well. Sandy closed down her mobile, switched on the headlights and began the drive.

"Just hope our hotel's got a night porter," she told Roger, who nodded in his sleep.

Chapter 3

Most of the time the voices in Jane's head were so familiar they sounded like old friends nattering away in the background. Not particularly kind friends. Generally they echoed the sort of catty remarks girls at her old school used to make about anyone just out of earshot who they'd previously pretended was their pal.

Jane understood the girlhood anxieties that made them do it. She'd done it herself. It was almost like a nervous defence mechanism: talk about them before they talk about you.

Some days it felt as if her whole life had just evaporated before her eyes. One minute she'd been young, the next this fag-ash Lil of a middle-aged woman stared back at her from the mirror.

And nobody, nobody, told her the truth. Not her mother, not Sandy, not the nurses and psychiatrists who'd allowed her to wallow for months - or was it years - before finally coming up with an apologetic: "We're sorry, we believe it's schizophrenia!"

Sandy had immediately joined a support group. Soon, she was breezily telling Jane not to worry…that schizophrenia affected: "One in 100 of us at some stage in our lives…" It seemed this was an episode; she'd get over it. Then Sandy had gone off to university, got married and eventually had a child. Meanwhile, Jane was still trying to get over it.

Of course, she'd long ago grasped the fact that her problems were far more physical than mental. The nervous breakdown had been real enough. The depression left in its wake was just some understandable, though totally irrelevant bonus ball. Although apparently not irrelevant to the doctors. It was the reason they refused to discuss her real illness. After all, officially, she was a psychiatric patient. Not that this excused her own mother, or Sandy, from continuing to treat her like a child, begging her to cut down on smoking when they already knew it didn't matter what she did because it was too late. Her heart condition was incurable.

Sandy just flew into a rage whenever Jane tried to explain how she'd personally overheard the doctors discussing her irregular heartbeat when they'd retired behind the hospital screens.

"They've already told us there's nothing wrong with your heart, or your blood pressure," she'd yelled.

Whoever she asked it was always: "Oh no, you must have heard them talking about somebody else, you're just a nutcase…sorry."

Jane knew her little sister was only trying to protect her. As one of the more authoritative voices in her head kept reminding her: *"Heart disease is incurable. It's just something you live with. For a while."*

It was a case of keep taking the tablets. Keep up the injections. Even when you're feeling fine, keep up the injections. Jane wondered if Sandy had ever considered Botox like some of her 'forever young' clients. She'd love to see what some of them looked like after years of her sort of injections.

Perhaps my bum's a vision of loveliness, she thought.

Grinding out her cigarette in a hand-painted Royal Doulton saucer she'd picked up at a car boot, Jane shoved back visions of the nightmarish locked ward where she'd been sent after the worst breakdown. After Bruce.

He'd been the sociology lecturer who had opened her mind to the world, earned her undying love, then ditched her as soon as the next set of first years arrived to inspect the campus.

It seemed Bruce's wife had always understood his light-hearted peccadilloes. Jane had not. Beneath her thin veneer of student sophistication she'd believed this was true love. That Bruce was her destiny. She believed it even on the morning she found herself teetering on the edge of a bell tower above a church where she and Sandy once went to Sunday school.

It was hard to know who'd been more frightened. Her, or the young curate who eventually managed to talk her down. He was probably a bishop by now.

Chapter 4

In Pau, the winding mountain road was almost deserted. Roger was still snoring softly as Sandy flicked through the radio channels until she found some soothing late night music on the BBC World Service. The baroque notes of Handel's Water Music seemed the perfect antidote to the heady African rhythms of earlier and it was so peaceful under the stars.

Finally warmed, she smiled at the simple pleasure of being able to casually pass on the kind words of this man with the thinning ponytail who wasn't her daughter's father. Roger was, she had to face it, more hip than her. There were flecks of silver in the hair pulled back from his temples and wrinkles in his face. But they were wrinkles full of laughter.

Sandy was always told her eyes were her best feature – a mesmerising turquoise according to one disgruntled business rival. Her hair was fair, with a little discreet help from her stylist, but somehow inconsequential. It was Jane's that had all the strength and vitality; just not Jane herself.

*****

I'm hardly old, mused Sandy, who was 43. So what if this man was a year or two younger – "Not the sort of information I'd reveal to a gorgeous PR woman..." he'd winked when they first met.

Sandy smiled to herself. It wasn't the sort of information Roger would reveal even when he qualified for a bus pass. He was incapable of growing old. At the office her personal assistant, Claire, had followed the progress of their old-fashioned courtship with vicarious excitement – before tactfully suggesting that if things were getting serious, perhaps they ought to get Roger checked out on the police computers. Sandy had been briefly offended by the well-meant, if slightly over the top idea. As an occasional supply teacher Roger already had clearance to work with children. Oh why was modern life so fraught with suspicions? Because it was, and perhaps we are all the better for being less innocent, sighed Sandy, blinking as the headlights of an oncoming car dazzled her. It was the first vehicle she'd seen on the road for some time.

Roger was a tender and sensitive lover who'd smiled and kissed her when they first got together and she confessed to being out of practice in the bedroom. It was through Bella's talent on the guitar that she'd met him. Now, whenever he came to visit, he always brought his own guitar so he could teach her daughter some new riff before dinner. Sandy, never the most confident cook in the world, loved hearing them tuning up together as she rang for pizza with extra pepperoni or a Chinese takeaway.

On the back seat of the car lay a gift-wrapped guitar strap featuring Bella's favourite band, The Slam, which she and Roger had chosen together.

After years of hard work, things finally seemed to be going right in Sandy's life. She'd built up her own PR company virtually from her back bedroom and now had fashionable offices in the city centre.

Last year she'd been named runner-up in the local businesswoman of the year awards.

Since then things had been going better than even she could have dreamed possible. Of course, she still rushed around too much – she knew that. It was the one thing her delusional sister was right about. Was half of it a reaction to the static life Jane herself led?

Dear Jane. All she'd done was fall in love with the wrong man. That had been the start of everything. The start of the illness, the start of the panic attacks and endless anxieties, the opening up of that yawning black hole that seemed to swallow her sister whole and from which she couldn't, or wouldn't, climb out.

"The more lifelines I try to throw, the more she resists," Sandy told Roger, who frowned as if he understood.

On good days, and after more than a quarter of a century, even Jane acknowledged the absurdity of always living her life as if she was in imminent danger of a heart attack. But she believed it anyway.

Taking a firmer grip on the wheel, Sandy remembered the latest hurtful letter, virtually word for word. It was almost funny. Jane was always good at expressing herself.

She'd written: "I don't know why you've bought me this cat. Animals are your thing not mine. Don't you think I have enough to do trying to look after myself without you and our mother going on and on about how I should eat more, smoke less, take exercise, do a computer course, learn French, start art classes....oh yes, and how about getting a job!

"Don't you think I feel guilty enough about being on benefits! And that doesn't mean I want you to put me on your payroll as a filing clerk. Unlike you and the rest of your celebrity-obsessed 'team', I don't actually care if I never get to meet Posh and Becks...."

After more ranting about the unwanted 'gift', Jane had concluded: "Perhaps it's you that needs something to love instead of..." What was it? Oh yes: "that guitar-twanging toy-boy you're wasting your time with."

As the starlit road stopped twisting upwards and levelled off, Sandy listened to the soaring music and reflected on how much of her own life she'd spent feeling guilty. As an imaginative and intelligent older sister, Jane had done so much to broaden Sandy's own horizons. Why now, when she was ill and her life so...so cramped, couldn't Jane accept help from those who loved her?

I'd never have got my maths O level without her, thought Sandy, yawning. With the benefit of hindsight, she understood now how she should have stopped confronting Jane during the early years of her illness. But that first breakdown had turned her sister into some sort of skeleton version of them both, all their girlhood fears strung-out, jangling on a pole for all to see.

Jane, Jane, it was such a waste... sighed Sandy, as her breathing became deeper, her eyelids began to droop, and she was gently enveloped in a plunging, floating sensation…that ended in a jarring, ear-splitting crash.

*****

After the grinding, smashing noise it was the screaming that upset Sandy the most.

The left-hand drive hire car had turned a complete 90 degree angle as it skidded into a tree, smashing Sandy's head hard against the door as the airbag streamed out to trap her startled face sideways on, looking straight at Roger. Gradually the mechanical noise subsided to a hiss of engine parts as silence descended on the vehicle and Sandy noticed the lightest flickering of snow started to fall all around. But the screaming, that horrible gut-wrenching hysteria carried on as she looked at the blood pouring from Roger's leg and tried to reach across to him. Her arms wouldn't move. He was slumped, face-forward, in the soft pillow of his airbag, which was a red colour. Why was his red and hers white?

The Mondeo had crumpled like a concertina against a tree and, from its small plateau, pointed down towards the festive lights of Pau. The windscreen was crazed at the front but clear at Roger's side where, incredibly, a figure seemed to be shouting and gesturing.

The car radio had somehow jumped channels and loud reggae music was pounding out. Closing her eyes, Sandy opened them again to glance across at Roger to catch his reaction.

Knock Knock, Who's There?

As she tried to turn her face the screaming took on a muffled tone. Roger's eyelids flickered. But he did not wake up. Her head was throbbing.

"I'm going to die," she realised, labouring for breath. "I'm going to die. Please God let someone look after Bella. I'm so sorry...."

Chapter 5

Anorexic chef Ray had punched holes into a cardboard box so that Jane could take the kitten back to the RSPCA home where Sandy had found him. She didn't mention the animal's imminent return to Wendy. If the warden wanted a cat she could get her own. Jane would even donate the cat flap. But not Mr C. He'd have a better life away from Fruitcake Towers.

She was standing at the bus stop just up the road from the house when her mother drove past without noticing her, peering as she always did over the top of the wheel as she indicated far too early, looking for the turn into their drive.

In the distance Jane could see the bus coming and was tempted to carry on waiting. She hesitated, then, without knowing quite why, walked back to the flat, carrying the box.

Did she secretly want a row? She didn't really know. These days she had so little to say to her mother who she noticed, for the first time, was beginning to look like an old lady.

"Ah, there you are. What's in the box?" asked Mary absently, as she locked the car and watched Jane walking carefully up the driveway.

"Evening," said George, who was just coming out. Neither of them commented on the fact that a more appropriate greeting might have been "Morning."

"The cat."

"I see."

Knock Knock, Who's There?

If her mother had bothered to recount how she'd also tried to dissuade Sandy from this latest "get-well-quick" scheme, Jane might have offered to switch the kettle on. Mary didn't say a word. But appeared to want to come in anyway.

Reluctantly, Jane allowed the complaining Mr C to climb out of his box. As soon as they crossed the threshold, the cat shot back out of the door, no doubt making a beeline for Wendy's flat.

"Well, what is it now, mother!" said Jane, who was always surprised and sometimes a little ashamed by the level of her automatic reflex aggression.

"Do you think we could have a cup of tea?" asked Mary.

"You haven't noticed what I've done to the place," said Jane, filling the kettle with petulant reluctance. "Not that I ever wanted to come here - surrounded by people I've nothing in common with. Even our so-called caretaker has only been out of school five minutes. And she's got about as much tact as a rhinoceros."

Mary found the very familiarity of her daughter's rage almost a comfort. Normally they would have gone at it like hammer and tongs within minutes of being alone together. Mary could never understand why Jane wouldn't try harder at some office job, even a therapeutic one. Jane always started so well and her new employers would think they'd hired a cut-price wonderwoman. Nobody understood that it was keeping the routine, day in, day out, that always let her down.

As Jane squeezed a tea bag between two mugs, she gradually became aware that the bristling tension normally surrounding these visits was only coming from her. Something was desperately wrong.

Astonishingly, Mary said gently: "Why don't you have a cigarette?"

"Mum, what is it?"

Mary dissolved into tears. "It's all right, I think it's going to be all right…I've had some very worrying news. Sandy has been involved in a car accident in France. She's got some sort of head injury and they're keeping her under sedation. I don't understand how serious it is yet – they're speaking French. I mean, of course, they are French. A nurse was trying to explain in English but her accent was too strong.

Jane sat down and tried to light up. Her hands were trembling uncontrollably. Even so she couldn't take in the words her mother was saying. Sandy couldn't be ill, she was never ill.

"It's me that's sick." Jane formed the words in her mouth although no sound came out.

*****

"They think she fell asleep at the wheel," sighed Mary, going round to the kitchenette and carrying back the two weak mugs of tea. After taking a sip she began to cry again.

"I've told her, I've told her – and your father was always telling her before he died – she's always running around too much."

Then Mary began talking quickly, too quickly for Jane to follow all the details. It seemed her mother was booked on a direct flight to Pau in three hours time. Bella had already been told the news by her head teacher – simply that her mum had been involved in a car accident and was being treated at a hospital in France. Jane was needed to pick up Bella and keep her for the night – perhaps a couple of nights.

There'd been no point in being too explicit with the head about Jane's 'unusual' living arrangements. He was bound to raise objections and there just wasn't the time to explain.

"We both know that Bella will need to be close to one of us at the moment and so that has to be you," said Mary. It was important to be positive. Everybody had to think positively.

Somewhere in the jumble of words, Jane noticed that pony-tailed Roger, Sandy's boyfriend, was now being referred to as her fiancé. It seemed one of his ribs had pierced a lung during the crash and he had suffered a broken leg. Even so he was expected to make a full recovery. Sandy couldn't be moved but she needed familiar faces around her.

The French doctors said it wouldn't be a good idea to let Bella see her mother at the moment. She might be frightened by the facial injuries, which were described as largely superficial.

"Jane, I've got to go. Bella will be able to get a bus from your flat to school and I just haven't got time to call anyone else. I've already talked to her on the phone and she says she'd like to come and be with you. The teachers think it's best if you just send her to lessons as normal until we know more.

"Jane please, please try to be strong. Don't be ill right now, we all need you to be strong, especially Sandy and Bella."

Mary stood up and put her arms round Jane. "Come on, get your coat. It's best if you pick her up now and bring her back here to wait for more news. Do we need to clear it with that caretaker woman? All right, you do that. I can drop you off at the school on my way to the airport."

*****

Bella's eyes were puffy and her nose was bright red from rubbing with a disintegrating piece of tissue. As soon as she saw loveable, crazy Aunt Jane waiting outside school, she burst into a fresh outbreak of tears.

Awkwardly, Jane hugged her niece and thought about all the times in the past when the two of them had played endless games of snakes and ladders. She'd have to buy another box. There were some playing cards somewhere in the flat. Perhaps she could teach Bella whist. No – neither of them would be able to concentrate. This wasn't happening. She was ill, not Sandy.

Except for the period after her husband died, Sandy always bounced through life. Even after Tom, she'd eventually picked herself up and coped.

It was Jane who'd begun the nosedive into another relapse and ended up back in hospital.

Knock Knock, Who's There?

She'd seen it coming and at first tried to get help. But it was the usual Catch 22 situation. If you're well enough to know you're ill, you're not really ill at all.

The doctors had taken not the slightest bit of notice until Jane took to wandering the streets late at night believing she'd made arrangements to meet Indiana Jones. When anyone expressed doubt she explained, pityingly, that of course she knew her date was really with Harrison Ford. It was the one time Sandy hadn't been there like a shot with helpful suggestions passed on by her support group. Their father had made an appointment with one of the senior consultants. Much good it did him.

Patient confidentiality meant the doctor refused to discuss details of a case without the express permission of that patient. Jane had been up on the ward, practising handstands at the time. The new medication hadn't kicked in yet.

That was the first time she'd ended up on a locked ward. It was all so long ago. She knew Bella remembered her Grandad - but not her own father, from whom she'd inherited red hair and most of her freckles.

Jane had still been in therapy when grieving Sandy had gone on to sort out a loan from some listening bank or other and opened her own public relations business. Now she had pop stars and footballers on her files and was forever off to literary lunches and champagne receptions. It seemed she was good at her job too. She'd already ghost written the life story of an inarticulate goalkeeper who'd once been married to someone off Eastenders.

*****

"We'd better go back to my flat," Jane told Bella. Together they waited for the bus, hand-in-hand, like crestfallen children cast out from a birthday party. Neither of them knew what to say, so they said nothing.

When they reached Peacehaven Mansions, Ray was waiting outside Jane's door. He was holding a casserole dish full of beef stew, with dumplings. The cat was mewing around his legs and Bella, who had started crying again, immediately swooped on the creature and swept it into her arms.

"Oh, you did keep Mr C – Mum said you might give him away…" said Bella, pressing her face into the soft fur.

"Of course not," said Jane, lighting a fag and glancing across at Ray, who for some reason was smiling. She fumbled in her bag for the key and let them all in. Ray immediately took charge of the situation, switching on the two-ring cooker and wedging the casserole dish into the tiny oven.

"We really need microwaves in these flats," he said, putting on the kettle.

"I'm out of fags," said Jane. "Bella d'you think you could nip up to the shop for me?"

"Don't be daft, they won't serve her," said Ray, who'd been explaining to Bella how he used to work on cruise ships and be number two chef at the Hotel Metropole. "I helped train that Robbie Wotsisface who's always on telly," he added.

"Was he a really great cook, even then?" asked Bella, her eyes opening wide with wonder.

"Well, he turned up for work in dead fashionable gear and always had clean fingernails," blustered Ray. He remembered all too clearly trying to teach the chronically lazy, skintight jean-wearing, future celebrity chef how to thicken sauces, make Caesar salads and dress crab. The lad had moved on to an even more prestigious hotel shortly before Ray decided he was sick to death of food and was leaving. It hadn't helped that he'd been found drunk in the larder. Again.

Chapter 6

After a restless night Bella emerged from Jane's bedroom at 7am to find her aunt curled up on the settee. Her mouth was open and she was snoring loudly. A full ashtray was on the table next to the settee.

When she went to the bathroom Mr C rushed out and mewed enthusiastically. Bella searched in the cupboard for a tin of cat food and began hunting for a tin opener before realising it was a ring pull can. A marketing slogan on the top read: "Is there a £1 million voucher inside?"

There wasn't. But there were more slugs in the cat's bowl. Bella shuddered and emptied the food into a clean dish. Jane had woken up and was watching her blearily.

"Hey, I don't let the cat eat off my best plates," she said struggling up, then flopping back down again.

"I've got to get to school," said Bella.

"Oh, have the day off – nobody will expect to see you today," said Jane, turning over.

"But I want to go – they might have some news of Mum. The head said he would tell me as soon as he heard anything."

Suddenly Jane was wide-awake and bristling. "Oh, I see – you mean they'll tell him but not me – the lunatic!"

"I don't know....won't Grandma ring you as well....what about the
answer phone?"

Jane and Bella stared at each other. Jane knew if the phone had gone off right next to her ear last night she wouldn't have heard it. Bella walked slowly towards the instrument, picking up the receiver as if it was cut glass. Her hand shook as she held it to her ear. The dialling code hummed.

"Nothing," she said. "I'm going to school."

"Wait, wait, I'd better come with you," said Jane, struggling to get off her makeshift bed and in the process knocking the ashtray onto the floor.

"I'll get it later," she said and grabbed her coat. She didn't mention breakfast.

Outside it was freezing. Buses were wheezing their way up and down the main road, people were coughing and small children were wailing. It seemed nobody wanted to go to work, or school. Except Bella.

"I've got my pass but you wouldn't have any money I could take for lunch, would you?" asked Bella apologetically.

"Oh, oh yes," said Jane, fumbling in her coat pocket. She pulled out £5 then a handful of change. Bella glanced at the £5 note but picked out the change from her aunt's hand.

"Are you sure that will be enough?" asked Jane, trying to keep the relief out of her voice. She didn't get her Disability Allowance until Friday and hadn't got a cigarette to her name. She was already planning to go back and pick over the dimps. It wouldn't be the first time. At least her flat was on the same route as Sandy's house in the suburbs.

"I'll just get off here then tonight, shall I?" said Bella as the bus spluttered to a stop. "If I don't hear anything."

"Yes, come back here – I think I've got some frozen lasagne in the fridge," said Jane, putting out an arm to hug her niece, awkwardly. She noticed that the hem on Bella's school skirt was hanging down.

******

But when Bella returned, at 4.30pm, it was to a dead house. Nobody at Peacehaven Mansions appeared to be at home. She banged hard on her aunt's door. Then banged harder. And waited.

At least the news was encouraging. Grandma Mary had rung the school and Bella was allowed out of a history lesson to hear that her mother had briefly opened her eyes and seemed to be responding to treatment. The doctors had been worried about the risk of swelling to Sandy's brain but seemed happier now.

Her grandmother had borrowed a mobile phone from one of the nurses and Bella had spoken directly into her mother's ear…Grandma said it didn't matter what she said. Just the sound of her voice would help Sandy to slowly come back to consciousness.

Turning up the collar on her blazer, Bella wandered round the overgrown garden and wondered whether yelling would bring Aunty Jane? Or Ray, or George…or someone? It might be June but the sun hadn't been out all day.

"Hey, hey, is anyone there?" she shouted trying Ray's door. An old man shuffling by on the road glared up the drive with disapproval as Bella hammered harder and harder on the door. The cold air made her breath come out in clouds. They couldn't all be out. Renee hardly ever went anywhere. Which one was Wendy's flat?

*****

It was Mr C who emerged first, stretching luxuriously and purring round her legs. The cat flap slapped open in the front door. Then a muffled yell from inside gave Bella hope. It was starting to rain when Jane, her hair sticking up like an aged punk rocker, finally stumbled to the door and yanked it open.

Wafts of hot air and stale cigarette smoke billowed out. Inside, the electric fire was on full blast and an old black and white film was flickering on the video. On the draining board there was a line of dirty cups and some baked beans on toast congealed on a plate. Aunty Jane, still befuddled with sleep, looked round apologetically.

"Sorry for the mess," she said, "It's these tablets I take, they make me sleep all the time. The others are the same. It's just the way it is here. Do you want a cup of tea?"

Bella nodded and wondered whether there was any hope of something to eat.

"Grandma rang you, didn't she?"

"Oh yes, it sounds fine. Told you your Mum'd be all right. Sandy's as strong as a horse – always has been. She'll be back home in no time. That

Roger seems to be doing all right as well. He's in the same hospital – different wards.

"By the way, when did he become your Mum's fiancé?" In her anxiety Bella had forgotten to ask Gran about Roger.

"Don't know," she shrugged, finding it hard to turn away from the fire. Tentatively, she asked: "Is there anything to eat?"

*****

Jane rang everybody she could think of in a bid to find somebody more suitable than her, to look after Bella. Most people were shocked to hear of the accident but lived too far away to be of much practical support.

Two of Sandy's closest friends did offer to have Bella after Jane told them straight how she wasn't well enough to cope with her niece - the house was full of mad people – the child wanted feeding all the time – she was coughing with all the smoke and needed to keep regular sleeping hours.

"You know what I'm like, I'm not reliable and we'll all get into trouble having a child here. I know Wendy won't be happy when I tell her about it."

One friend said she would be able to have Bella next Wednesday but could Jane just hang on or find somebody else for the weekend because she needed to keep her mind clear for a two-day interview for a new job?

"There's still a glass ceiling out there for women," she explained, by way of an apology.

Knock Knock, Who's There?

The other friend lived ten miles away in a village on the other side of the city. She wanted to rush round straight away and said she would get Bella a temporary transfer to her own daughter's school until the situation resolved itself.

Jane was surprised when she heard herself saying: "No," that wouldn't be necessary.

"Bella will be better off staying with familiar friends at her own school. I guess I can cut down on the fags, a bit," she added, replacing the receiver and wondering what the hell she was playing at.

A nicotine patch and 40, instead of 50 a day, had been her all-time record.

*****

In the end there was nothing for it but to introduce the child to her fellow flatmates. As well as Ray, who lived round the back, there was slug-disposer George, multi-pierced Amanda, who used to sleep rough in London, sad Jim, who was clinically depressed, Winston from upstairs, and Renee, who suffered from agoraphobia and was slightly deaf. This was probably a good thing as her flat was right next door to slug and heavy-metal lover George, whose bedroom was up in the house's imposing circular turret.

Caretaker Wendy had flowering tubs and a hanging basket outside her door at the front. This was an effort to detract from the wheelie bins and weeds clustering round the side driveway. Wendy hated it when they called her the warden.

*****

"Knock, knock, who's there?" Winston asked Bella when Jane took her up to his flat.

"I'm Bella Bradstock," laughed Bella, who was cuddling Mr C in her arms. She'd hardly put the animal down since arriving at Peacehaven Mansions.

"Hi cat," said Winston, his thick glasses glinting as he reached out to tickle the kitten's ear. "He seems to be settling down well."

Resplendent in a Hawaiian shirt and a pair of carpet slippers, Winston seemed oblivious to Jane's meaningful glances and proceeded to show Bella the front-page newspaper story he'd had framed and hung on his wall. It was dated five years earlier and all about him being sent to prison.

Later, when they went back downstairs and began doing a jigsaw on the breadboard, Jane grumbled: "Course, even hardened criminals don't seem to get sent down these days. Not that Wint deserved to go. Nobody really knows why he's in here – far too cheerful. He hears a few voices – must be old comedians – but he's a lovely bloke. His mother brought him to England from Jamaica when he was about nine. Wint's never hurt anyone but himself."

"Why did he go to prison then?" asked Bella, searching the board for a bit of blue sky.

"The court case was because he went into Woolworths with soaking wet feet and nicked a dry pair of socks. He put them on, there and then, in the middle of the store. Later he got annoyed and threw a brick through a window at the Citizens' Advice Bureau."

"Why did he do that?" asked Bella.

"Why do you think? Because after his arrest he wanted some advice and the place was always closed.

"Apparently even the magistrates apologised for having to lock him up. They made some excuse about a probation report being late and there not being a spare bed in some secure loony bin that weekend. Poor Wint was ill and needed some help. But they ended up remanding him in prison for a week surrounded by some real hard cases."

Jane took a deep drag on her cigarette.

Bella said: "I've never been inside a courtroom. Is it the same as on telly?"

"When d'you think I've been to court? I'm ill, not a criminal!"

"Sorry," said Bella, not looking remotely contrite. The two smiled at one another.

"But if he only pinched socks and broke a window why did he get on the front page?"

"Oh because when the magistrates went out to consider their verdict Winston's Mum...Betty - that's her name, was in a right state. And the flaming lawyer who was supposed to be on Winston's side just ignored her and started chatting about a golfing weekend with the man from the prosecution!

"It was only some reporter on the press bench who took any notice. She could see Betty was upset and tried to cheer her up by explaining how most people only got a conditional discharge for that sort of trivial first offence.

"Course when Wint was sent down his Mum went berserk. This young girl ended up taking her out for a cup of tea and borrowing some old photograph that Betty carried in her handbag. Next day there it was, headline news: 'Mental Patient Jailed for Stealing Socks'…some rubbish like that. It was all true though."

Chapter 7

Feelings about Fruitcake Towers had always run high among some of the regulars at the Queen's Head. Many still believed the council had blurred the truth and successfully conned them into accepting madmen and women in the district. And while it was true most of the newcomers seemed nothing more than mildly eccentric, others were right psychos. You only had to see them in the street to know they had a screw missing.

It made Brian and Ian Beddows bloody angry. The brothers had grown up in the district of Cranmere and both had young kids. Brian was a warehousemen and regular writer of letters to the evening newspaper. If it was the last thing he did, he'd get that half-arsed, politically-correct, effing liar of a ward councillor out next time. Ian was younger, a bricklayer and the pub's reigning pool champion. Usually, he agreed with Brian.

Nobody could accuse the brothers of not being hard-working members of their West Midlands estate, which was mainly a mixture of 1950s council houses, now mostly in private ownership, a few pretty pre-war cottages and a newer development added during the 1970s near the site of the old chemical works. People said there'd been some funny-looking vegetables pulled out of the gardens of the "new houses" over the years, but nobody took too much notice. Brian remembered how their dad had earned good money at the works, before it closed.

After they married both brothers bought homes on the modern estate and, although the area had slipped a bit as jobs got harder to find, Brian and Ian still felt a strong sense of community. At weekends they didn't mind lending a hand to some of the old dears living over the back in the original 1930s cottages who always had problems maintaining their properties. Ian was particularly handy at mending broken sash windows and reluctant to accept a tenner "for a drink" when it was thrust upon him.

He knew the old ladies thought they were treating him and didn't realise how much the price of a morning's labour had gone up. Not that he minded. Their houses were full of interesting stuff and dated back to when Cranmere had been a rural backwater. One old boy had been the gardener up at the big mansion on the main road. He was as angry as they were when it was converted into Fruitcake Bloody Towers.

One way or another the elderly were gradually moving out. Brian had been an active member of Neighbourhood Watch until he fell out with the co-ordinator for pussy-footing around.

The two brothers knew what was what. They took their sons to play football every Sunday and Ian had successfully deflected his youngest daughter's interest by forking out for horse-riding lessons instead. He didn't like bruises on girls. They took their wives out every Saturday night, played in the pub pool league on Tuesdays and met up before the traditional "last orders" time every Thursday.

Knock Knock, Who's There?

"You look after your own," said Brian, sinking his third pint after a successful pool game. "Why should we be expected to look after every Tom, Dick and effing perverted Harry?"

While Ian got the drinks in, Brian glared across at the stick-thin geezer in the corner who, between gulps of beer, seemed to be carefully studying each peanut from a bag before sticking it in his gob. You could tell the bloke had already had a right skinful. God knew what was going on in his head. Yesterday he'd been laughing with some young schoolgirl. Him and that other old bag who always had a fag in her mouth.

"Look at 'im – effing alcoholic. He'd do anything for a bloody drink, " Brian muttered to Ian and the other men at the bar.

"Come on, he's not doing any harm," put in a soft bloke Brian remembered from school. "Council said they've never done owt violent."

"Got kids of your own now, Wayne?" he asked, already knowing the answer was no.

Glaring across at the drunk in disgust, Brian knew he was deliberately getting off his head. He was a man drinking to forget. Someone capable of doing anything if the moon was full or the wind changed direction. Those smug council buggers would tell you any old rubbish. Well, it wasn't his kids that were going pay the price for care in the bleeding community.

Chapter 8

In the hospital in the French mountains the hours crawled by. Mary had drunk more machine-made coffee and lemon-flavoured milkless tea than her system could cope with. She seemed to be on a continuous loop between Sandy's intensive care room, the refreshment counter and the loo, after which she looked in on Roger's ward before starting the whole cycle again.

The nursing nuns who ran the place were kind, if incomprehensible, and she had to make sure she was awake when the consultant who spoke the best English was on duty. The monitor beside her daughter's bed continued to bleep, encouragingly, and Sandy herself had started to have fleeting moments of consciousness. Her lovely face was horribly swollen and she had two black eyes.

By contrast Roger's ribs were healing well. His leg was in plaster but he seemed comfortable enough. He told Mary he was passing the time listening to music and trying to do a bit of composing. Every day he always asked how Sandy was and had been wheeled through to her ward on a couple of occasions.

On the practical side he'd recorded Mary and himself speaking into a decrepit radio cassette he'd borrowed from one of the nurses and set it up to play continually in Sandy's room. With great embarrassment, he'd also had to borrow 350 Euros from Mary to get the crashed hire car moved off the mountain road and into a garage. The insurance company said it looked like a write-off and wouldn't pay the hire company until they could interview Sandy.

"I hate having to ask you for a loan," Roger told Mary, "I gave up teaching to be a performer and just don't have lots of spare dosh splashing around these days."

Mary already knew about Roger's former teaching job. She hadn't dared to tell Sandy but once the two of them seemed to be making a go of things she'd plucked up the courage to ring his old school in Brighton and asked to be put through to the head teacher.

Sandy really hadn't had all that much experience of men apart from her late husband who'd been dead ten years. Like many clever people she wasn't always blessed with an overabundance of common sense. And in spite of what she did for a living, she always thought the best of people, insisting life would be impossible if we all didn't occasionally rely on the kindness of strangers. A quote from some classic book she liked, apparently.

The headmistress in Brighton had been frosty at first when Mary had explained she was enquiring about a Mr Roger Bailey. Fortunately, she was also a mature woman who after a few minutes understood where Mary's questions were coming from and that she was a concerned grandmother, not just any old nosy member of the public.

"No," she'd said, wearily: "There were no problems during Mr Bailey's time with us – he's obviously a talented musician and was quite an inspirational teacher."

It seemed Roger was simply not the most reliable of staff members. "He left us in the middle of term, with very little notice, to go off on tour with some band," said the head, adding: "I hope he's happier in what he's doing now. I suspect some of our female members of staff rather miss him – bit of a charmer."

Not for the first time, Mary wondered what her younger daughter was letting herself in for with this man. But the taped messages and songs, playing on the radio cassette next to Sandy's bed, were comforting, and thoughtful.

*****

Drifting in and out of consciousness, Sandy was still re-visiting the scene of the crash. At first she frequently woke up screaming and there was terror in her eyes as she tried to work out where she'd heard that noise before. Then she remembered and slumped back, closing her eyes in pain.

Sometimes Sandy was dimly aware that her mother was by the bedside. But where was Bella? What had happened to her daughter? No. That was it, Mum said Jane had Bella. Jane would take care of Bella.

But Jane was ill.

"Jane is ill," she kept trying to tell the silent nuns. But they didn't seem to understand her.

Knock Knock, Who's There?

"Jane is ill," she told her mother's face. But her mother just dabbed at her with a damp flannel and told her not to worry.

Then Roger was there, smiling, and he was telling her not to worry as well. But where was Bella? Who was looking after Bella? Oh yes, Jane. Bella would look after Jane.

No, she was getting confused, Jane had to look after Bella. But Jane was ill...

*****

Before she drifted back into unconsciousness, Sandy glimpsed the old-fashioned cassette player on the bedside table. It triggered so many memories. Her mind floated back to when she was sixteen and had just finished O levels.

Jane had come home from university. Jane was ill. Jane was ill then. She came home from university because they said she'd had a nervous breakdown.

It was late spring or early summer. A concerned woman from pastoral services had telephoned and suggested Jane might want to consider taking a year out.

Their parents had been baffled. It seemed the wife of a senior lecturer had complained that Jane was harassing her husband, following him around and standing for hours outside their home. The couple's **two** springer spaniels had taken to howling throughout the night.

Delicately, the woman from pastoral services had explained how first year students often found it hard to settle down when they were away from their families for the first time. It was a question of maturity. Jane had completed most of the first year of her sociology degree successfully. But it was now clear she wasn't well and some essays were long overdue. They were prepared to consider keeping a place open for her next year – perhaps on a different course.

As soon as Jane arrived home she was prescribed anti-depressant tablets by the family GP. The doctor also made Jane an appointment at the local psychiatric hospital although the date set wasn't until the following month.

Despite the happy pills, the old Jane just didn't seem to be there any more. She was haggard and far too thin.

Sandy stayed at home as her friends embarked on a post-exam round of non-stop parties. It wasn't only Jane who needed her support. The guilt had started back then. Because Sandy had known something about the affair with Bruce the Boffin – as Jane had once playfully described her lecherous lecturer in a letter. Gleefully, Jane had told her about how much she fancied Bruce, and how he appeared to be pursuing her. She'd known he was a married man but he'd explained he and his wife led separate lives.

In the same letter she'd raved about sociology being the most fascinating subject she'd ever studied. How Sandy really ought to consider it as an option at A level and drop one of those Mickey Mouse media courses she kept on about.

As an idealistic teenager Sandy had been scandalised - this lecturer was old and married - but sworn to secrecy. Jane said if she breathed a word to either parent she just might feel the need to tell Dad about Sandy's recently acquired taste for trying "herbal" cigarettes.

"I should have said something, I should have said something..." mumbled Sandy, tossing all her blankets off the hospital bed. She'd been too scared to ever puff on more than half a joint and went off normal tobacco in a fortnight after deciding chocolate was cheaper and more satisfying.

At home it was impossible to penetrate the gloom that descended over the whole house. Jane was like a stranger. She hardly ate, didn't want to wash or go out anywhere and kept constantly hovering around the telephone in the hall. Often she stabbed a few numbers in very quickly, listened for a while, then hung up and ran upstairs. They all heard her sobbing in her room.

Once, Sandy had quietly pressed the re-dial button. All she got was an automatic voice repeating: "This number is no longer available...."

Just when everyone was at their lowest ebb, a flash of the old Jane would bubble up, almost from nowhere. It was always during unexpected moments like the time Dad dragged an old tape recorder down from the attic and they'd listened to their childhood voices pretending to be BBC announcers.

Jane had laughed for the first time since she'd come home. She listened to her schoolgirl self trying to do a commentary on a football match where she kept getting the players' names muddled. She'd kept having to issue: "No, it isn't…oh yes it is" corrections in pantomime-style before finally bellowing "Goal!"

The tension in the house had evaporated for a glorious half an hour. It's going to be all right now, it's going to be all right now, Sandy remembered thinking.

Her sense of relief echoed down the years, the feeling so strong that her lips formed the words, silently, as she slept in the French hospital bed. It wasn't all right. An hour later they'd found Jane standing in the hall, grinding her cigarette into a plate of sandwiches and stabbing numbers into the telephone again.

*****

The English-speaking consultant told Mary and Roger that it would be at least another week before they could except to see real signs of improvement.

"She's still blocking out the accident," she explained slowly. "It's going to take time but we are very…optimistic… that Mrs Bradstock will recover."

Leaning heavily on a pair of hospital crutches, Roger seemed chastened. "I keep forgetting that

Sandy is, was, a Mrs. She's always just lovely Sandy with the beautiful eyes to me."

"She and her late husband were very happily married," said Mary, with a hint more acid in her tone that she'd intended. She'd just had to loan Roger another 100 Euros.

This man with the ponytail had been a shoulder to cry on over the past few days. He was just so different to Bella's father, who'd been a solicitor. True, he seemed to care about Sandy all right. But he was so…frivolous, careless of life and responsibility. A bit younger too. Though he did make Sandy laugh - something she hadn't done that much of in recent years – as well as doing wonders for Bella's guitar playing. And the child wasn't resentful of her mother's romance. She seemed genuinely fond of this, well, ageing hippy.

Chapter 9

During the first week of Bella's stay in Peacehaven Mansions, Jane managed to avoid telling Wendy about her new lodger. She knew the warden would find out soon enough. In the meantime, a less haywire pattern of living began to evolve at the house.

Instead of spending all afternoon in the Queen's Head, Ray squeezed what cash he could out of Jane, added a bit of his own from his essential drinking fund, then went to the market to buy bacon, cheese and as much fruit and veg as they could afford.

Personally, Ray never touched fruit but providing food for others was what he was good at. And it gave him pleasure to see the child tucking in – he even found himself eating a few leftover potatoes and gravy. Ray noticed Jane developed a taste for the odd kiwi fruit if he included one in the new eco-friendly 'bags-for-life' the Co-op was pushing as an alternative to the plastic variety.

Once Jane got up, grabbed her purse and actually went to the market with him. But the fags on offer were so much cheaper than the off-licence up the road she ended up bulk-buying a bigger supply than normal.

Pensioner Renee, who the others nicknamed The Watcher because she spent hours gazing out of her upstairs front window, had burst into tears when she first saw Bella. It wasn't until two days later, when Bella was borrowing milk, that Renee explained how she'd at first thought the 12-year-old was her long-lost daughter come to find her.

"It was silly of me really - she'll be five years older than you, nearly 18 now," said Renee. "But when you came up the stairs with Jane, I wondered, just for a minute, whether you might be her."

It turned out that quite late in life Renee had given birth to a ginger-haired baby daughter although her "stick-in-the-mud husband", was not the father. Their three teenage sons had been disgusted and sided with him.

For the sake of the marriage, and her boys, Renee had agreed to have the little girl adopted. Soon afterwards she'd been admitted to hospital after pushing another woman's pram home from the shops. She'd been treated for post-natal depression but after being discharged her marriage had broken up. Now her grown-up sons rarely visited.

"She'll be 18 in a few weeks," repeated Renee. "And one day she's going to come looking for me."

While she continued to wait, and watch, Renee agreed to adjust the time of her afternoon nap so that she was always awake when Bella got back from school. As soon as she caught sight of the youngster getting off her bus, Renee went into her bathroom and banged with her walking stick on the ceiling of Ray's flat, directly below. Even if Ray had enjoyed a session at the Queen's Head he still managed to get up, splash his face with cold water and go round to hammer on Jane's door. It wasn't long before she loaned him a key to her flat. Everybody knew Jane slept like the dead.

When warden Wendy did find out about Bella she was far from happy with the situation. She certainly didn't think a young girl should be stopping in what was essentially a halfway house for former psychiatric patients. But when she telephoned social services there was nobody in to deal with the matter. Typical really – they were always off with stress, on holiday, or on some course or other. She'd written a formal letter to make sure nobody was going to blame her for the situation, even if it was a family emergency.

*****

Mr C basked in the glory of the new living arrangements. The cat had never had so much attention in its young life. Bella doing her homework at the kitchen table was a soothing, non-comatose presence who hugged and absently tickled him under the chin. Jane refused to allow the animal to sleep in the bedroom and now that she occupied the lounge settee at night, she always locked him in the bathroom. There were worse places. And if Bella felt upset about her mum, she sneaked him out and onto the bed.
The news from France continued to be encouraging. Mary had bought herself a mobile phone. Now even Jane's shrill calls to 'get well soon' were regularly blasted across the English Channel and directly into Sandy's right earlobe. Mary always said the pitch of Jane's voice had the

most impact on Sandy, who nearly always opened her eyes.

At the weekend Bella took Jane and Ray back to her house to collect more clothes and check the mail. There was a ton of Get Well cards and some bills. Jane and Ray pointed out these weren't even red ones so could be safely ignored. Bella picked up her guitar and her mum's laptop, then started to cry.

"It's all right, it's all right," said Jane, "She'll be back soon."

"But why won't they let me see her?"

Jane tried to explain. "I don't know, Mum says she looks so battered and bruised and there's really nothing to do but sit there. You know what your mother's like about having days off school. As soon as she wakes up we'll get the next flight."

"Are you coming?" snivelled Bella.

"Well, I will if you want me to."

"Have you got a passport then?" asked Ray.

"Oh, bloody hell. I don't know where it is – do they still do visitor ones?"

"You must be joking!" said Ray. I'll make some enquiries. There must be some sort of emergency provision."

Their conversation reminded Bella to root through a drawer and collect her own passport. Then she began crying again.

Chapter 10

Unlike Jane's slugs, Roger Bailey had been a very welcome alien invader into the lives of superwoman company director Sandy, and her daughter Bella. Although no formal decisions about the future had been made, Roger's occasional overnight stays had become more regular over the past two months - something Bella had never experienced before.

And finding shaving cream and men's deodorant in their bathroom verged on the exotic in a household that had been exclusively female for so long.

Bella's father had died of a rare strain of meningitis two days before her second birthday. Sometimes she looked at old photographs and pretended to recognise the bearded man wearing a bumblebee-striped rugby shirt, if only to please her mother. The truth was Bella's only real memory was of a big person with a wide smile, a booming voice and a scratchy face. Her Dad died before anyone realised that he was suffering from much more than a persistent cough.

The numbness that surrounded Sandy at that time could so easily have engulfed her. It was only the support of her parents, and the day-to-day routine of having to care for a toddler, that had pulled her through. With hindsight Sandy also put it down to the resolute toughness she had acquired from years of riding on the emotional roller coaster of Jane's illness.

Knock Knock, Who's There?

Bella remembered that on her third birthday she'd been whisked off to an early morning children's film and stuffed with ice cream by her late dad's less familiar, and rather posh parents. Bafflingly, they'd tried to explain it was a year since her Daddy had gone up to live in heaven with Jesus. Bella just thought it was her birthday.

In the afternoon she'd been released into the company of Aunty Jane, Granny Mary and her adored Grandad Bill and they'd all gone to the zoo. Her mother had stayed in bed all day.

Bella also remembered the first signs of her smiley old Mummy coming back. It was when she'd handed over a still-wet painting after her first morning at playgroup. Things got better after that. Except Aunty Jane had to go back into hospital for a bit.

Grandma Mary and Grandad Bill called round most nights to read her bedtime stories before going to visit Aunty Jane. Bella asked to go with them when they left for the hospital but she wasn't allowed. Slowly, her aunty had got better and started helping out in a charity shop from where she loaned lots of jigsaw puzzles for Bella. As soon as the two of them completed the picture the puzzle went back on sale. Except for one particularly difficult one of the Forth Bridge that took so long they couldn't bear to break it up. Sandy had it framed.

Bella must have been seven or eight when Jane went back into hospital with what everyone said was "another relapse". Listening to the grown-ups arguing it seemed as if it was all the council's fault.

They didn't have enough money to pay the teacher of a pottery class Aunty Jane enjoyed going to every week. The council said she could do the same lessons at the old people's home up the road from Grandma's house. But Aunty Jane had got really upset because she wasn't old.

That was the first time Bella had been allowed to visit the mental hospital. Sandy had got special permission on the grounds that she might cheer Aunty Jane up. Bella still remembered the long, green tiled corridors in the hospital and how slowly her aunt had walked as she came up the ward towards her. Then she'd smiled and they'd had a game of Snap which made Aunty Jane laugh, even though she kept losing. Most of the other patients were glued to the telly. One man kept laughing uncontrollably. Aunty Jane said she wouldn't mind taking the same tablets.

Sandy kept on visiting although by then she'd thrown herself back into work. Before Bella was born Sandy had held good jobs with two well-established PR agencies and still had lots of contacts. Widowhood galvanised her into action by the basic need to keep up the mortgage payments on their stylish home in semi-rural but still edge-of-the-city surroundings.

Bella loved the house and never knew there'd been a time when they might have had to give it up. The place was big for the two of them but it backed on to the far edge of a cricket pitch where in the mornings she could look out of her bedroom window and see rabbits.

Knock Knock, Who's There?

There was also a riding stables up the road and a tennis club where she and her mum had made new friends, even though most players took the game a lot more seriously than either of them did.

Setting up her own business from the spare bedroom meant Sandy had zero overheads. Even better was the fact that she'd remained personal friends with a couple of minor celebs from her last agency.

These were not minor celebrities any more. One had become a judge on a television talent show and the other was an award-winning, but penniless actress with the Royal Shakespeare Company who regularly arrived at their front door in flamboyant anguish.

To keep working for the prestigious, but poorly paid RSC, the actress desperately needed to endorse a few products on television and do more wildlife voiceovers. Sandy had promised to investigate hair shampoo, and perhaps tampons.

Within weeks the press attention she'd carefully cooked up for both 'starter' clients, attracted a string of new ones. The only setback had come when her own father, Bella's adored grandad Bill, died six years ago. He'd just got worn out, Mary said.

To cope, Sandy, who always thought she was tone deaf, had joined her mother in becoming a member of the Golden Lining Ladies Barbershop Chorus. It turned out to be a corny but a comfortingly large consumer of leisure time for both widows. Many weekends were spent singing in seaside towns where Bella could play all day in the sand watched over by kindly choir supporters not required at rehearsals. Sandy found the other women, although mainly older, were also a great giggle on lonely Saturday nights.

*****

Bella had always boasted to Aunty Jane and Grandma Mary that it had been her who'd really brought Sandy and Roger together. She'd introduced them a year ago after he'd been the adjudicator on her Grade 5 guitar exam. Bella knew she'd done pretty well and so it seemed perfectly natural when leather-trousered Roger - who wanted directions back to the railway station - asked if the lady waiting outside was her mum.

Performing for a test was like taking to the floor on an ice rink. It didn't matter how much practice you did, you could still fall flat on your face. In fact Bella had only made one stumble during her set pieces. And Roger – Mr Bailey as he was then – explained that it was the way she'd quickly corrected herself and carried on playing that was the key to success.

"We all make mistakes," he'd winked, pen poised to make notes on his clipboard.

Sandy had offered the music teacher a lift to the station and when his train was delayed they'd agreed to have a coffee with him.

It turned out "Rog," as he liked to be called, was a guitarist and occasional keyboard player in rock bands, a jazz band and a 'covers' band that performed in the styles of lots of different groups.

"Who's your favourites? he asked them. "Arctic Monkeys, White Stripes, Sting, Oasis, The Jam...I go back a long way," laughed Rog.

Bella had kept a discreet silence about her mum's true musical tastes - otherwise they might never have hit it off. When Sandy asked how her daughter had done in the exam Roger put on a funny voice and joked: "Lady, it's more than my job's worth to say." He didn't have to. All three knew Bella had played really well.

And that had been the start of Sandy and Roger as a couple. At first the invitations to concerts had been to both mother and daughter. Roger would be playing at some county festival or backing a singer Sandy half-remembered from the past. He would get them tickets and suggest they meet him after the gig. Inevitably some of the concerts were late and so Sandy would go alone. Bella had been a bit put out at first – after all she was the serious musician in the family. But not when she began to realise how much happier her mum had become.

They'd also introduced Roger down at the tennis club where the professional coach – who Bella suspected had always had a thing about her mum – scathingly told them their new 'friend' played the game like a "mad horse" full of high kicks and impetuous leaps. It was embarrassing – but so funny.

Once Roger got free tickets to see REM who he insisted were still one of the 'ultimate' live performance bands. He said Sandy had to be ready early so they could stand in the first few rows. Bella wasn't too upset about missing that one but she advised her mum not to get too close for fear of being crushed in the '"mosh pit". Roger had roared with laughter.

"REM's fans will all be even older than me and your Mum! They won't mosh. They'll be too busy picnicking on quails' eggs and bottles of Chardonnay."

Most weekends Roger was working but when he came to dinner during the week he never forgot to bring his guitar. He also brought Sandy flowers and perfume. She brought him an electric toothbrush for when he stayed the night. Roger confessed to Bella he'd never spent more than £2 on a toothbrush in his life. During the first few months of knowing them, Roger grew, then shaved off, what Sandy described as a Van Dyke-style beard. Then he'd started to let his hair grow longer. Sandy told him he looked sexier with short hair.

"Got to keep changing my image, depending on which band I'm performing with. Just a trick of the trade," he grinned.

Sandy had begun to make discreet adjustments to her own appearance. Slightly shorter skirts, higher heels and a bit more mascara. By then she'd already left the Golden Lining Barbershop Ladies' Chorus and begged Bella and Mary never to mention it. All three understood the transition from local solicitor's widow to lead guitarist's girlfriend was going to take some image makeover even for a PR woman.

But the prize was Roger. Sandy wondered whether she'd have been quite so attracted if he'd worn his hair in a ponytail when they first met. Then she smiled and asked herself who she was kidding. It was seeing Roger on stage that really wowed her. That was where the real Rog lived.

She understood now that he was the ultimate performer, one minute bending into his electric guitar to produce the most amazing riff, the next dancing to the front of the stage to engage with the audience, then he was back, musically flirting with some soul singer, getting the best out of them.

His hair might be going grey but his raw musical sex appeal raised everyone else's game as he thrashed out yet another breathtaking set of what Bella assured her mum were brilliant improvisations. Nearly every performance was a minor triumph.

"It's like acting," Roger told Bella one night, his skin still glistening with sweat.

"You bounce off each other and get feedback from the audience. Every night it's a different crowd out there, a different mix of people. There's nothing like it for giving you a buzz. Wait until you play live."

The idea that she might ever be good enough thrilled Bella so much she was walking on air for days.

By the time she'd received her delayed Grade Five guitar pass with Merit - distracted Roger hadn't filled in the form properly – he and her mum were an item. And there were definite advantages.

Roger seemed to have a genius for getting free tickets for good indie bands playing locally. He and Sandy often dropped Bella and one of her school friends off. In the two months leading up to the French trip Bella realised she was spending slightly more time at her grandmother's house than before. Not that she'd really minded. Roger played a lot at weekends so she could usually rely on spending Saturday nights with her mum.

But the days of climbing into her bed so they could read together on Sunday mornings were gone. Because Roger was usually there.

Chapter 11

Jane was not impressed with Roger Bailey.

"I'm sorry, I just don't like him," she informed Sandy after being introduced to the first man her sister had taken seriously in ten years.

"Well that's a relief then!" said Sandy, hurt, but knowing only too well that Jane was an irrational law unto herself.

"What's a man of his age doing with drainpipe jeans and a hair bobble? I know he's a bit younger than you but not that much younger!"

"Aunty Jane, he plays jazz. They're all like that," put in Bella, determined not to be left out of this important conversation. Rog made her mum laugh. He made her laugh too, and gave her tons of help with the guitar. Within three months she'd passed Grade Six with Distinction although this time Rog explained he wasn't allowed to adjudicate because he was "seeing" her mum.

Jane said: "There's something shifty about him, I can't put my finger on. He's not as patronising as you but I'm sure he's smirking behind my back...and he doesn't like me smoking, you can see that."

Suddenly Sandy snapped. "Oh shut up Jane! Up to last year he's spent half of his adult life playing in bars so thick with smoke and dry ice you can hardly see both ends of the stage! You're being absurd – or jealous."

Bella still winced when she remembered the row that had erupted.

Barbara Goulden

They hadn't seen Aunty Jane for nearly a month.
Sandy had bought her the kitten, as a peace
offering. By then her aunt had moved into the new
flat and at first said she couldn't handle the
responsibility. But it was the cutest kitten in the
world with lovely smudges of ginger, white and
brown – tortoiseshell, her mum said.
After a lot more ranting and raving followed by a
full rundown on the latest state of her irregular
heartbeats, Jane had reluctantly agreed to a
period of trial ownership.

*****

Jane knew she was often unkind to her sister
without any real cause. Still, it did irritate the life
out of her the way Sandy would sweep into any
dilemma she was facing with an instant answer.
She was always so confident and always so damn
bossy.
I know she means well, Jane remembered in her
more charitable moments. And she cares about
me, just like I care about her, and Bella, and our
dear, exasperating, mother. Not that even Mary
could see the dangers of this Roger bloke. God,
he was dodgy, if ever anyone was. Why was it
only she could see it?
When she wasn't worrying about her health, or her
next date with a psychiatrist – it was rarely the
same one - Jane's voices had become very vocal
on the subject of dodgy Roger.

Knock Knock, Who's There?

"AND I'M NOT JEALOUS!" she shouted at the new kitten, which jumped several feet into the air then hid behind the sofa. Sandy might be a hard-headed businesswoman but she was an innocent abroad on the emotional front. True, she'd done all the right things at university, including 'not' falling in love with a lecturer. But then she'd married Tom - whose job it was to believe every Legally-Aided story that came through his door - and they'd spent six or, was it seven, years trying to have Bella? Not that the child hadn't been worth the wait.

After all those years with a dual income and no kids – what did that make them? Oh yes, Kinkys…no, Dinkys…they'd put the deposit down on that dream house in suburban splendour. Dream for them anyway.

Meanwhile, I'm sitting in this shoebox waiting to die, thought Jane.

"We've all got to die sometime…." said a singsong voice in her head. It was a girl's voice. Jane recognised it as one of her regulars. She decided to ignore it.

Sandy knew nothing about the treachery of men.

"Of course, you know far too much," another voice. A man this time. Someone she hadn't heard from before. Or was it the family GP?

"Toooo much, what do you know Jane? Toooo much…." The man had started chanting.

"Come on, Jane, What do you know?" repeated the girl in her head.

"She knows nothing," said the man, *"she's ill, waiting to die."*

"When will you die, Jane?" asked the girl. *"Tell us, tell us when you're going to die?...."*
Jane knew the voices were not going to let her go – she began rifling through her emergency supply of familiar videos. Sandy had offered to buy her a DVD but she didn't want the bother of new technology.
"It's no use ignoring us, we won't go away," whispered the girl. She was such a familiar tormenter, Jane knew she would go on all night given half a chance.
Where was her Clint Eastwood video? Oh no, Ray must have borrowed it.
In the drawer there was a young Dustin Hoffman in The Graduate, Robin Williams in Mrs Doubtfire, Judy Garland in The Wizard of Oz...no, no, it gave her nightmares.
"I bet you do fancy that Roger bloke yourself," said the girl, now in wheedling tones. *"Is that why you're always going on at Sandy? She really likes him...he really likes her...."*
The kitten had just ventured back out from behind the sofa when Jane shouted: "He's bloody dodgy!" It darted back, mewing pitifully.
Aloud, and forcefully, Jane said: "It's my job to worry about my sister, not yours".
"That's right, you should be worrying about your heart. How many beats did it miss last night?" said the man. *"Not that anybody cares..."*
"Nobody cares, nobody understands," said the singsong girl. *"Is it because she's a loony?...."*

Knock Knock, Who's There?

Jane began humming loudly to herself as she came across Kevin Costner in Waterworld and slammed him into her VCR.

"Come here cat," she ordered, banging a cushion behind her head and forcing herself to sit back in the room's single armchair.

The kitten didn't move. But after the film had been running for five minutes it crept out and pawed at Jane's skirt until she lifted it onto her lap. The voices in her head dimmed, though continued their background chorus. She was starting to calm down when the video jammed and Coronation Street came on instead with Deidre Barlow saying: *"Of course, Jane's had that heart murmur ever since she was a child."*

Ken said*: "Personally, I don't think she'll live long so she might as well carry on smoking."*

In the flat upstairs one of George's heavy metal bands began thumping out.

"Yes Jane, you might as well carry on smoking," repeated Kevin Costner's voice as the video suddenly untangled and the screen flipped back to show his co-star, Dennis Hopper, striking a match on board a wrecked oil tanker that was about to go up in flames.

Chapter 12

Eavesdropping on the stairs one night Bella had learned a lot more about Roger and his past life. It seemed he was so keen on her mum that he'd let the jazz band he belonged to go off on a European tour without him.

"Hot Jalapeno are good, but let's face it, they're never going to be mainstream," explained Roger. If only the girls from school could see him. He was wearing shades and designer stubble. He probably had a six-pack like the men in the Pepsi-Cola adverts. Not that Mum would ever say.

"I've reminded my agent I'm only an hour away from London. I won't be short of session work and, if things get tough, I can pick up some more supply teaching," Roger said.

It seemed he'd already taken on a temporary residency with a Sixties tribute band called "Who What." Her mum had been worried he was giving up too much but Roger said Who What was a 'regular earner' and there'd be lots of other tours.

"The Jalapenos have promised to keep my place warm when they come back. At the end of the day we're all individual players in that outfit – just have to keep at the cutting edge. Keep evolving. You know a lot of that stuff you and Bella watch on MTV is just some commercial spin-off from what happened first in jazz."

Her mother said what bands like the Jalapenos really needed was a rich sponsor.

"You said it," agreed Roger, who'd started to go on about the Renaissance of all things. He said the main snag in the fifteenth century was the artists were always told what to paint.

"Mmmm, I seem to remember the Sistine Chapel wasn't bad," laughed her mum.

"Mmmmm, and I seem to remember you might move in the same circles as a lot of millionaire football hunks who might want to model themselves on that well-known patron of the arts, Charles Saatchi."

Phew, thought Bella. Was he talking about Tracey Emin's unmade bed?

Then she heard her mum giggle something about keeping the music business closer to home. There'd been a lot more laughing and they must have opened a bottle of wine before Roger said: "Anyway, staying in this country will help me focus. I'll drink less and have more time to work on my own compositions....not to mention having more time to spend with a certain, wonderful new lady in my life...."

Ugh, they were probably kissing.

She was heading back upstairs when she heard Roger start talking about how he'd been married before to a woman called Elaine.

Her mum must have already known that because she wasn't surprised. Roger said the break-up was all his fault. Elaine had wanted a family when he just wanted to get out of teaching and run away to the circus! Bella didn't know what he was on about until he added: "I mean the musical equivalent of the circus. Childishly perhaps, I just wanted to do what I'm doing now. Play in a band - lots of bands."

Roger said back then there was no way he'd been mature enough to take on the massive responsibility of being a dad. It made Bella want to cry and wish she wasn't listening. But somehow she couldn't creep away.

Anyway, it seemed his wife had met someone else. Roger was glad and they'd gone their separate ways. It seemed he could see now how he'd avoided being straight and just made a mess of things. And the more he taught kids how to play, then watched them starting their own bands and playing at school dances, the more he wanted to grab his own guitar and jump up on stage and join them.

"How sad's that?" concluded Roger ruefully.

But it was what he said afterwards that remained forever engraved on Bella's memory.

"And some of those kids were so good, you know – like Bella. I've told you what a promising little player she's becoming. She's got that spark – the bit you can't teach.

"I don't know whether she'll want to make music her life, like me. Let's face it - I'm not exactly dripping in Porsches. Perhaps it will just be a great hobby. Either way, she's definitely got ability."

There seemed to be the sound of more kissing. After that the pair went on to talk about going away on holiday together. Her mum said she'd always wanted to visit the Pyrenees.

As she floated back up to her room Bella thought about the dizzying possibilities of a future that included Roger as her stepfather. How one day he might let her play in his band if somebody rang in sick. Only in an emergency, of course.

Chapter 13

Jane had cooked a meal. It was on the table when Bella got back from school. A stew, with microwaved jacket potatoes.

"What do you think?" she asked. "I went to the market at lunchtime and look - I even bought apples and oranges and some more kiwi fruit. Our favourites!" Bella lifted a fork tentatively to her lips. It's very…tasty," she said, instinctively knowing she should measure every word with care. "What sort of meat is it?"

"Stewing, or braising steak – not that I know the difference," replied Jane, who was wearing a new pair of blue and green parrot earrings.

"You know I used to quite enjoy shopping and snooping round the charity shops until the government stopped us having a rest in the nearest café."

"You mean because you can't have a cigarette with your cup of tea?" said Bella.

"Exactly. I practically stopped going out at all last winter. Anyway, by some miracle I managed to get some sleep last night so I was awake for ITV's This Morning programme. Ray's told me they do a lot on food so I watched them make this Dorset casserole and noted down the ingredients.

"I mean it could be I haven't got all the quantities absolutely right, but I can't be far off. And I asked the butcher how much meat Ray usually buys."

"It's really filling," said Bella, chewing stolidly.

Flushed with success, Jane went on to say how she was thinking about borrowing some of Ray's cookery books. The good news was Ray himself was actually eating a bit more these days. The bad news was he was also drinking a lot more. And still getting into rows with the regulars in the Queen's Head.

"I've told him to give it a rest – he doesn't need the aggravation. Even George's told him and busybody Wendy's told him. Trouble is, he won't listen."

Jane was still pondering the problem of Ray when there was a hammering on the door. Mr C sprang off the chair dragging Bella's school tie, which was caught in his claws. Jane peered through the spyhole in her door but really she knew, by the tone of the rat-a-tat-tat, it could only be Winston from upstairs.

"Knock knock, why did the farmer bury all his money in the fields?" asked the beaming Jamaican as she opened the door.

"I don't know…because he was a loony, like us," laughed Jane.

"Naw, he wanted richer soil!"

There was rarely any alternative to letting Winston in. Apart from occasionally thinking his flat was infested with rats he was perfectly sane. He'd always been a joker and since Bella arrived had taken to trawling the internet to update his repertoire. The sock-stealer and self-proclaimed jester of Peacehaven Mansions had the knack of lifting everybody's mood.

"Hi cat," said Winston, getting down on his hands and knees and crawling round the back of the settee to stroke Mr C. The kitten couldn't resist coming out when he waggled the other end of Bella's tie.

Winston tickled the animal under his chin, then stopped stroking it and asked: "Do you know why the chicken crossed the road?"

Mr C surveyed Winston carefully, assessed there was no food, or any other advantage to be gained from this over-familiar visitor, then raised his tail and scrambled back onto the chair, where he immediately started a furious fight with the tie still attached to his back leg.

"He really looks at home now," grinned Winston.

"He's not stopping," said Jane. "And why....?"

"Why what?"

"Why did your latest chicken cross the bloody road?"

"No need for profanity," sniffed Winston, who'd been brought up as a regular Sunday worshipper. "I've forgotten now. Anyway, what did the tie say to the hat?"

Glad of the distraction from the stew, Bella decided to join in.

"I don't know, what did the tie say to the hat?"

"You go on ahead and I'll hang around. A head! Get it?"

"Do you want a coffee?" asked Jane, pursing her lips and smiling in spite of herself. Bella giggled.

"Wouldn't mind. What you two up to tonight?"

Jane shrugged, filled the kettle and opened a new packet of cigarettes. She got a spare mug down from the cupboard and fished a dry cream cracker from a dusty-looking biscuit jar.

Knock Knock, Who's There?

"Haven't got any sweet biscuits but d'you want some margarine on this?" she asked Winston.

Although she'd been friends with plenty of Asian girls at school, Jane had never really known any West Indians before moving to Peacehaven Mansions. On good days Winston's infectious smile and hopeless jokes were irresistible.

He'd told her: "White doctors are always wary of black patients. They think we're going to punch them. 'Course sometimes we do," shrugged Winston, who personally wouldn't hurt a fly. It was the sock-stealer's personal charm that had kept him safe during the week he'd spent at Her Majesty's pleasure.

"You know Ray's drinking - more than ever," said Jane. "He's going to say something in that pub and end up getting into a fight."

"I know, but what can we do?" said Winston."

"Can't you get a doctor?" asked Bella.

"Wouldn't do any good," said Jane. "He'll only say Ray has to get so low that he's prepared to ask for help. God, he's an idiot!"

"Well, we wouldn't be here if we was all Einsteins," put in Winston. "Which reminds me, what did the scientist say to the lunar module?"

"Oh shut up Winston! There's nothing wrong with my brain and apart from losing your way as a stand-up comedian there's doesn't seem to be much wrong with yours," asserted Jane. "Anyway, even Bella understands it's a physical illness with me."

Bella carried on chewing. If Aunty Jane was laying down bait she wasn't going to rise to it. It was a trap she'd seen her mum fall into all too often. She could already re-run the familiar scene in her head. How many times had she heard her exasperated mum say: "But Jane, you know the doctors have already given you a full medical examination. Physically, you're as strong as an ox..."

Only for Aunty Jane to reply: "D'you think the doctors will admit the truth to me? I know how my heart races at night...and so do they. They just won't come clean about their real diagnosis yet they all know I can't go on much longer. It's you who can't accept the facts when they're staring you in the face. The truth is I'm living on borrowed time. I could have a heart attack at any moment..."

Instead of following the well-worn route of questioning her aunty's reasoning, Bella polished off most of her meal, hid the remains under a cabbage leaf and reached for her guitar.

She said: "Shall we have a game of snakes and ladders?"

Chapter 14

If anyone had asked Jane to complete a customer satisfaction survey on her experience of psychiatrists, the ratings would not be particularly high. One or two she'd liked over the years. But to all doctors she'd feigned an aloof indifference. It was no good letting them get too close. Some had jocular bedside manners which might suggest they wanted to be friends – "we're in this together, fighting your illness" – but you just couldn't allow yourself to be misled.

Most of them did want to get you better, Jane didn't deny that. Though it was hardly a relationship of equals when one person had the power to lock up the other. Or order a stronger drug regime which brought horrible side-effects in its wake.

Jane accepted that she'd had a nervous breakdown when she was 20. However, she was totally convinced the doctors had misdiagnosed her subsequent long-lasting depression and developing heart disease as schizophrenia. Their refusal to tell her the truth – no doubt because she was so "mentally fragile" – had been responsible for a whole series of "revolving door" hospital admissions throughout her twenties and thirties. These days she forced herself to accept the cocktail of medication they'd prescribed to keep her mood "stable".

Like all the other tenants of Peacehaven Mansions, Jane's fear of psychiatrists was based on their ultimate power. Her poor opinion had its roots in the humiliating periods of trial and error she'd endured while they were trying to get the balance of long-acting anti-psychotics right. Too strong and you were virtually comatose. Too weak and the voices might crowd in and overpower you with their negative messages of misery.

Then, when they finally got the drug balance right and you'd listened to everybody else's woes at group therapy, the hospital discharged you with some largely 'mythical' programme of aftercare. This might involve follow-up visits at a local day centre, a place on a computer-training course, even some therapeutic work placement in a local office or shop. Whatever was arranged, it never started straight away. There was always a gap. You came out of hospital willing to give life another go…and there was nothing. Because the day centre was temporarily oversubscribed; the computer course was halfway through and you had to wait for the next one to start; some admin officer was away and no paperwork had been completed for the work placement.

Always there were two, three, or four weeks where you were back living in the same situation that had driven you mad in the first place. In Jane's case that had been back at home with Mary, who was fond of reminding her what an intelligent 'girl' she was and how she could be doing more to help herself. Kicking her heels, waiting for the prescribed rehabilitation remedy to start, Jane had decided more than once that she'd rather be mad than continue taking such powerful medication. Sometimes it could leave her with blurred vision or trembling hands.

And her decision seemed right because at first she always felt far better when she stopped popping the pills. Her energy levels would go up and her mind become more focused. She might have a whole week of remembering that she was still a young woman who had beaten back the voices; whose heart disease could be identified and cured...that it still might not be too late to meet someone and have her own little baby.

This surge of euphoria would start to wind down during the second week. It would continue to drop, lower, and lower, until she reached rock bottom. Usually it was her mother, or Sandy, who rang for help when Jane took to her bedroom and refused to come out.

Her depression could go on for months. And often there was no way back without being readmitted to hospital and going through the whole trial and error business again, knowing you were a failure. It was one reason the monthly injections were better. Although you still had to remember to swallow a few multi-coloured side-effect tablets if you wanted to stop the trembling or the blurred vision. Since moving into Peacehaven Mansions Jane realised that it wasn't just her - hardly any of them kept regular hours. They woke at different periods of the day and night, which meant the times they actually took any side-effect pills could vary dramatically. She'd already heard Jim threatening to give his medication a miss after getting the shakes.

Only a month ago she'd told him: "Look Jim, I've not had to go back into that place for nearly three years now. Try and hold on a bit longer – see if you feel any better next week."
Wendy was trying to persuade Ray to go into a drying-out clinic. Winston didn't recall when he'd last seen his psychiatrist although he did remember offering the man   his favourite feed line: "Doctor, doctor I feel like a pair of curtains…"
"He didn't tell me to pull myself together, just asked whether I was all right for money – you know getting enough Disability Living Allowance," said Winston, scratching his head.
Nobody could remember when Renee had last seen anybody more senior than the charge nurse at the outpatients' clinic. Like Amanda she seemed virtually well. And Jane always thought it was a waste of taxpayers' money sending George to see a shrink. Everyone in the house could have diagnosed his state of mind by the volume and choice of music he played.
Thinking about her last three years of non-admissions, Jane grudgingly supposed that the latest in her long line of consultants must be getting something right. After the perennial "How Are You?" this woman had been the one to suggest she moved away from her mother and tried living in a flat on her own. Even though it turned out to be a disaster, it was during this short spell alone, with nobody else to blame, that Jane developed some inkling of her personal 'red lights' - warnings of a major depression ahead.

Curiously, the consultant seemed almost pleased when Jane announced she wasn't coping. The place in semi-sheltered Peacehaven Mansions had followed. Of course, even this better-than-average doctor still flatly refused to discuss the fact that in 1980 Jane had personally overheard one of her predecessors discussing the dangerous deterioration of her heart.

"We've gone over that before," the psychiatrist said, her head tilted to one side and the suggestion of a smile playing about her lips. "All I can tell you is there's nothing on your notes.

"Now, let's talk about your schooldays. Were they happy?"

Chapter 15

At last Bella was allowed to fly out to France for the weekend. Despite Ray's efforts, Jane's passport could not be renewed in time so Bella resigned herself to travelling alone. She didn't mind. Jane had a win on a scratch card so she ordered a taxi to take her and Bella to the airport. Mary did the rest, including asking for a stewardess to keep an eye on Bella as an "unattended minor". When the child landed in Pau, Mary was there to meet her in a hired car.

Grandmother and granddaughter wept. But it was okay. Sandy's level of sedation had been lowered and they could make out some of the things she was murmuring in her sleep. Yesterday she'd asked to see Bella.

On the journey from the airport, Mary did her best to prepare her granddaughter. But it was still a shock for Bella to see her mum attached to a drip, her face puffy and bruised and a monitor bleeping constantly by the bed.

"Mum, Mum..." cried Bella.

Amazingly, Sandy slowly opened her eyes and, as if from somewhere very far away, she'd whispered: "Sweetheart..." then drifted back to sleep. As Bella sobbed Mary reminded her of what fantastic progress Sandy was making and how much better she looked than a week earlier.

"The doctors are really pleased with your Mum," explained Mary, speaking slowly and gently.

"She's drifting in and out of consciousness but she's coming back to us. It's the shock. Right now these drips and things are to keep her quiet so she can build up her strength again. It's going to be a while yet lovey, so we've just got to stick with it."

They sat silently for a few minutes before Mary added, absently: "Thank goodness for the holiday insurance, that's all I can say. "These hospital bills could have bankrupted all of us. Roger's cover ran out days ago – course he'd only taken out the minimum. And your Mum's secretary has been marvellous – sorry, personal assistant I'm supposed to say. She's certainly earning every penny the business pays her. So are the rest of the staff, they're all so loyal and supportive – I think your Mum's been a really good boss."

"She will be again, Grandma," said Bella, smoothing back the hair from her mother's hot forehead.

Later, Bella went to see Roger who she found rocking his head violently in tune with some music on an iPod. His greying hair, freed from its elastic band, was swinging around his shoulders. Bella could see one or two of the other patients on the ward frowning in disapproval.

Still worried about her mum, she was glad to see that at least he was looking almost the same - except for some boldly-striped borrowed pyjamas. As she watched him fingering an imaginary air guitar Bella knew Roger was too much of a child himself to ever qualify as a real replacement dad. But he was so full of enthusiasm for…well, everything. Off-stage he could be a bit theatrical and he looked more his age. But he was still cool - and he really did seem to care about her mum.

"Bella! Great to see you," called Roger, as he swung his head round, fingers still strumming, and finally noticed her. Pulling the ear-piece out and throwing an arm round her shoulders, he said quietly:

"Your Mum's a lot better, you know that don't you?"

"She spoke," said Bella.

"See, she'll be out of here in no time. And guess what? I'll be out of here next week – they say I'm well enough to come home. At least I think that's what they're saying....I'm going just as soon as that gorgeous mother of yours wakes up."

He grimaced. "Might have to start doing some supply teaching. The lads aren't back from Europe yet so any multimillion-pound recording contract they might have picked up will still be on hold."

When Bella looked baffled, Roger winked and asked how her practising was going. For the rest of the weekend she stayed glued to her Mum's bed in a private room. Her classroom French came in handy as the nurses kindly put up a camp bed while Mary, who looked worn out, spent two nights at a nearby guest house.

"I've got my mobile on at all times," she told Bella. "The nurses know to ring if there's the slightest change."

In the middle of the second night, Sandy suddenly snorted loudly, then jerked awake. Almost as if she knew this was only to be a brief intermission, she focused her eyes on Bella – who she didn't seem surprised to see – then began to whisper urgent questions about how she was getting on with Aunty Jane?

"Is your Aunty smoking too much? "Wouldn't you rather move in with a friend?" Sandy gabbled.

Before Bella had time to answer her mother slumped back into unconsciousness again.

"Mum, we're fine," Bella found herself shouting, helplessly, hoping that her words could catch up with her mother's drift back down into oblivion.

When Mary heard the news she was delighted. But the doctors said it could still be a long road to recovery, which reminded Mary that Bella shouldn't stay at the bedside too long.

"It's coming to the end of term and your Mum's going to need your help during the summer holidays. She won't like it if you miss too many lessons when all we can really do is wait," said Mary. Later that day, she added gently: "I think there's a flight tomorrow afternoon. And isn't it time you perhaps stayed with one of your friends?" But Bella felt closer to her mum when she was with Aunty Jane. Although secretly she did worry whether her aunty would remember to pick her up at the airport. It was unlikely she'd have any more scratch card wins to pay for taxis and the idea of Jane staying on the airport bus for more than an hour, without being able to have a cigarette, would be a challenge. Perhaps she'd send Ray, or Winston?

Sandy didn't wake up on Bella's last night but when Mary arrived next morning there was a further brief surge of clarity. And before Bella left to catch her flight, Roger had another of his inspired ideas. He borrowed an acoustic guitar from one of the hospital porters and he and Bella used the microphone from the computer in the day room to make their own cassette featuring some of Sandy's favourite tunes. Even Mary was yanked in at the last minute to add her "Get Well Soon" message to the finished tape.

Leaning on his walking stick, Roger used terrible French to instruct an awestruck young nurse to play the highly-distorted recording as often as possible. As he left to hobble painfully back to his own ward, Bella couldn't help smiling. Roger had such a showbiz presence that the French girl was left wondering whether he was actually somebody famous who she should be running after to ask for his autograph.

Mary said Roger would be following Bella back to Britain within the next few days. "You know, if you don't want to stay with a school friend why don't you and Aunty Jane go back to your own house and wait there?" she added. "I'm sure you'd be so much more comfortable."

But Bella felt she was used to Peacehaven Mansions now. And she had a key – although Aunty Jane had made her promise never to use it when Wendy the warden was around.

Even without asking, Bella knew her aunty would refuse to go home with her. She'd always complained their tree-lined street with its well-tended front gardens was full of nosy neighbours asking too many questions.

Roger said he could always collect some of his things then go and stay at the house to make sure everything was okay. Bella realised her grandmother didn't know quite how much of Roger's stuff was at their house already. The idea of him living there without her, or Mum, felt a bit funny. She remembered a conversation she'd had with her mother a few days before she and Roger went off on the holiday.

On one of their Saturday nights in, Sandy had confided: "You know I was wondering about asking Roger to move in with us. Though of course, that very much depends on how you feel about it."

Grown-ups were funny, reflected Bella. Did her mother think she was going to suggest they got married first? Sometimes she felt like she was the adult and her mother the child.

Chapter 16

After Bella flew home, Mary was left to gaze through the hospital window at the brown and white French cattle, endlessly chewing the cud. Her mind wandered randomly over the past three decades. Every time she looked back at Sandy, lying in the bed, she heard herself whispering: "Why you, why you?"

Sandy had always been so careful in life, so keen to do what was right. She'd already lost her husband and had tried so hard throughout all the years of Jane's illness. Despite all her ability to track down support groups, and her dazzling business acumen – where had that come from? – Mary suspected that Sandy was still in denial about her big sister. Only now was she beginning to realise that perhaps Jane might never return to her old self. That perhaps Jane now was as good as Jane was going to get.

The girls' father had been the same. Always thinking his clever first child could simply snap out of it if she'd try; pull herself together; all the usual cliches.

It was Sandy who found the schizophrenia support group after Jane was first diagnosed. It had proved a lifeline for both of them. Just meeting relatives of others with mental health problems, or hearing the survival strategy of some highly articulate ex-patient, had been inspirational. Not that everyone survived.

Over the years there had been at least ten suicides, some of them simply recorded as "open" verdicts announced by a coroner trying to be kind to distraught relatives. The handful of dangerous psychopaths dangling from the very top of the schizophrenia tree – the ones who hit the headlines - were rarely mentioned at meetings because they were so beyond most people's experience. They were the ones who gave the illness such a frightening reputation, even though it turned out the average weekend binge-drinker was far more likely to exhibit violent tendencies. The vast majority of schizophrenia sufferers hurt nobody but themselves – unless you counted the emotional damage they inflicted on those who loved them, sighed Mary.

Jane had always resented them going to the Schizophrenia Advisory Group (SAG). Even though they offered to drive her there so she could listen to the discussions, her sullen response had always been that SAG was just
a waste of time. Nothing more than a chance for sick people and their relatives to compete against each other to see which one of them had the hardest time of it.

In the hospital bed Sandy's breathing was even and regular. Mary smiled as she stroked her daughter's cheek. Aloud, she murmured:
"Remember what a blessed relief it was to find out we weren't the only ones with madness in the family."

Most of those who went to the meetings were parents, many were older than Mary and in despair about who would look after their "child" when they were gone. The 'children' in question could be aged anywhere from their twenties to their sixties. It didn't matter. They would always be children to their parents.

Actual ex-patients were in shorter supply but often made the most interesting contributions to the meetings. Especially when an expert speaker had been invited along to shed some light on the condition they knew all about from the "inside". Mary remembered how these former patients would often have the courage to challenge the experts and how one man, who confessed he'd always thought of himself as a "hopeless case", left a visiting psychologist in no uncertain terms about where he was going wrong.

The ex-patient, whose name was Steve, demanded to know why nobody in the medical profession seemed to take him seriously when he warned them he was getting his old symptoms back again. Even when his mother told the doctors they didn't believe her either. Every sufferer and relative in the room was familiar with the scenario. In the end Steve had shouted: "I live with this bloody condition every day….are you lot trying to tell me I don't recognise when my thoughts are getting illogical, or the voices are getting more insistent?

"D'ya think I want to go under? If somebody would just listen at the beginning of an episode then I just might save the NHS some money and not wind up in the loony bin. Again!"

Mary remembered nodding in agreement at these remarks. Jane was often so much more willing to accept help at the start of an episode - before she lost all insight into what she was saying or doing. Another time there'd nearly been a relatives' revolt when a smug-looking older psychiatrist told them they were not representative of the vast majority of relatives of schizophrenia sufferers.

He'd said: "Most people just get on with it and help the family member who's sick…they don't sit around beating their breasts and looking for members of the medical profession to blame."

He urged them all to remember it was the patients who needed the support; they just needed to calm down and keep things as normal as possible.

Sensing his words had not gone down all that well – a row of elderly mothers on the back row were practically foaming at the mouth – the psychiatrist swiftly departed saying he didn't have time to answer questions.

Surprisingly few brothers and sisters of patients turned up at SAG. Sandy had always been grateful when one or two did. Mary knew she was checking whether they too, shared her sense of guilt. Not that Sandy wasn't forever insisting that guilt was an illogical and unconstructive emotion. But it still helped when she realised the same feelings oppressed other successful brothers or sisters who had moved on with their lives, moved out, left the caring to those still at home.

You can only do what you can do, they all assured each other. Sandy told Mary every one of them felt badly about a mum or dad, usually a mum, who seemed to have become the focal point of their sibling's totally irrational anger.

Some people turned up at the group having never received a medical diagnosis of schizophrenia. They'd simply tapped symptoms into the Internet and come up with their own diagnosis, right or wrong. But as soon as they began talking about how they'd accidentally swallowed car battery fluid, or overheard the milkman talking about a national emergency involving contaminated dairy produce, Mary guessed they'd come to the right place.

One day a senior social worker based at the same day centre Jane sometimes attended talked about the need for families of patients, and ex-patients, to protect themselves if they were the primary carers. The social worker suggested the group think about the oxygen masks on planes which automatically dropped down if the aircraft lost pressure or hit turbulence.

She'd said: "Remember how the air hostesses always tell you that worrying bit about if the masks do fall down, adult passengers should fit their own over their faces before attending to the needs of any children.

"The same rule applies to you people," said the social worker. "Harsh though it sounds, if you don't look after yourself and your own needs then you will be in no position to look after those you are trying to help."

Chapter 17

The "ancien" radio cassette player – as the nurses called it – was left on constantly in Sandy's hospital room. Her medication continued to be reduced and there were longer periods of lucidity. The recorded voices of her daughter, mother and lover were so familiar and precious now.

The swelling on Sandy's face had reduced dramatically and she was differentiating night from day. When Mary arrived to sit by the bed   she always switched off the tape and re-tuned to the World Service so that Sandy could hazily half-follow plays and listen to quiz shows.

In the evening, when the younger nurses, who were not nuns, came on duty they switched to European pop. One 'golden oldies' programme played Abba singing *The Winner Takes It All.* Instantly, Sandy was back again in the summer of 1980 and her sister's first breakdown. She saw the face of her father, who by that August seemed to have aged ten years. Her mother had tiptoed round the house looking lost and exhausted. It had been a good instinct of Dad's, to dwell on the past. Old photographs, memories of music, films, seaside holidays, always soothed Jane.

But the rows had been terrible. Some flared up about nothing more serious than eating a meal or taking a shower. Others erupted from nowhere, taking everyone by surprise and always ending in tears, harsh words and slammed doors.

When Jane's appointment with the psychiatrist finally came round she was assessed and prescribed stronger anti-depressants. She was also given another appointment, in three weeks time. Sandy remembered her parents' confusion the first time a consultant explained how 'confidentiality laws' meant he really couldn't discuss an adult patient's case with anyone else – not even those who were trying to look after them. Their mother had given up her job, not wanting to leave Jane alone in the house all day. Both parents insisted they were "fine" when Sandy declared she was going to take a year out; not start her A levels until the following September. They might have put up more resistance except for the fact that Sandy had already done a two-week stint of work experience at what was the city's first free weekly newspaper.

She'd done well and Ronnie Graham, the editor of the Gazette, said he could offer her a six-month trainee placement while one of his reporters was on maternity leave. The hourly rate of pay was slightly less than she'd got stacking shelves at Tesco's on Saturdays, but the experience would be fantastic for her CV.

And the work was great. Sandy loved collecting the memories of old ladies celebrating their 100th birthdays – 101 and 102-year-olds were not out of the question – as well as covering carnivals and charity fun days. Bow-tied Ronnie seemed to spend a lot of time in the pub. Slowly, she came to realise that what she'd thought was a temporary piece of Elastoplast mending his broken glasses was actually a permanent feature.

Knock Knock, Who's There?

"I was what you might call tired and emotional, and fell over," explained the editor, who she'd heard some of the others describe as "a legend in his own lunchtime."

The news was nearly all good on the Gazette. It was such a relief from what was going on at home. Ronnie didn't do much training himself but Sandy learned most of what she needed to know from the paper's semi-retired gardening and rambling correspondent, John Shuttleworth.

The weekly paper was attached to the city's main paper, the Evening Echo, and had been quickly launched to see off competition from a rival 'freesheet' that was about to open for business and threatened to drain vital advertising revenue by offering cut-price rates.

As Sandy began to learn a form of shorthand, called Teeline, John told her of his glory days on the evening paper when reporters routinely took notes of court or council stories at speeds of up to 120 words a minute. They then sent runners back with copy to update the City Final. But the shorthand should only ever be back-up, said John. What Sandy really needed was to develop the knack of remembering the important bits of any story. Getting people to stick to the point and not go off on tangents all over the place was the tricky bit of being a reporter. Also everything tended to be black or white because there was little room for elaboration in a strict 350 to 500 word story count. Some news items had to be 'jacked-up' out of all proportion just because there was nothing good for page three.

After a while Sandy was allowed to cover the odd evening parish council meeting on the understanding that John would help her sort it out after finishing his gardening column.

"Not that anybody cares about local politics these days, the media's just obsessed with who shot JR!" moaned John. "You mark my words, this is the beginning of the end of serious journalism. I couldn't believe my ears when I heard the storyline from a television soap opera included in the BBC's nine o'clock news."

Sandy hardly liked to confess that she and her parents had become totally addicted to episodes of the Texas-based potboiler that spawned a craze for big hair and shoulder-pads. They relied on it as a complete switch-off from thinking, talking and worrying about Jane, who sometimes came downstairs to join them. They enjoyed Coronation Street too although Eastenders was just too hard-edged and depressing.

At work it was more golden weddings and ducklings born in unusual places that were meat and drink to readers of the Gazette. Sandy learned that pictures might be worth 1,000 words but all theirs had to be taken between noon and 2pm because that was the only time the weekly could borrow a staff photographer from the daily paper. She was also given her own patch to cover – a fairly well-to-do commuter village on the outskirts of the city where she cycled to meet the licensee of the local pub. She wasn't old enough to go in and have a drink but arranged to meet the landlord at the back door for a chat.

Knock Knock, Who's There?

He was one of the regular "contacts" passed on to Sandy by the reporter who was on maternity leave. It seemed she'd enjoyed a pint or two before she became pregnant and had helped him spearhead a campaign to try to save the local post office. This had failed but the landlord was still a good source of gossip and the Gazette was becoming increasingly popular. Partly because children only had to win a colouring competition or come first in a local cross-country race to appear in the paper's Grassroots News section.
Especially if their proud mum or dad could supply a picture.
On the Evening Echo hotshot real reporters like Jack Grady handled all the hard stuff like long court trials and hospital waiting list scandals. Sandy was accepted by the young graduate trainees, although sometimes, when she heard them discussing the best way to handle a "death knock," she doubted whether she was cut out for journalism. It seemed they had to go out and knock on the doors of homes where somebody had actually died in a car crash or accident at work.
It all sounded intrusive and terrible. Yet very often bereaved people were desperate to talk to somebody…have some record of the tragedy. Reporters would come back to the office carrying whole family albums of photographs. And Sandy realised that despite the intrusion, journalists like Jack always tried to find something good to say about a person who had been taken ill abroad, or killed in a motorway pile-up. Even when a door

was slammed in his face, he worked hard to find a neighbour willing to be quoted on how the deceased had once mended their car, fed their cat, or just seemed to be a generally decent type. The majority of deaths were due to road accidents or industrial injuries. But sometimes it was clear that a person who had jumped in the path of a train was mentally unbalanced. Their lives were written up in just a few short paragraphs. They were the sort of stories that really frightened Sandy.

Chapter 18

Back at Peacehaven Mansions, things would have been okay if depressive George upstairs hadn't moved into a manic phase at the same time as Ray shifted his drinking into a higher gear.

Miraculously, Jane had remembered to pick Bella up at the airport. She'd dressed in her smartest, only two-sizes-too-big navy jacket, matched it with a white pleated skirt and pinned on a pair of spiral sunburst earrings. She'd also made careful preparations for the 90 minute bus journey including making sure she arrived at the stop early enough to be able to smoke five cigarettes down to their tips.

In her oversized white shoulder-bag were not only 40 cigarettes but a jumbo-sized bag of pear drops, a nasal spray and some nicotine chewing gum which she hated and would only chew in the direst emergency. The voices were bad throughout the journey and her heart was hammering by the time she got off the bus.

It wasn't until she saw Bella's lovely little face, looking a bit lost at the Arrivals barrier, that Jane realised how much she'd missed the child.

"Mum's getting better," said Bella.

"I told you she would. Strong as a horse Sandy - always has been," said Jane, hugging her niece awkwardly before bustling her out of the terminal building and round the side for a few more frantic puffs.

Unfortunately, this meant they missed the first flight bus home and there wasn't another for an hour and a half.

"I didn't think you'd be able to make the journey," admitted Bella.

Like a conjurer, Jane solemnly rolled up first one sleeve, then the other, to reveal two nicotine "Quit" patches, one on each arm.

"I probably need to nip into the Ladies to renew them," she admitted, asking Bella to see if she could check the timetable. They'd finally got back to the flat sometime after 11pm.

Exhausted, Bella had only just dropped off to sleep when she was practically blasted out of bed by the sound of pounding rock music. The thumping was coming from above and involved a singer repeatedly yelling what sounded like "Purple Maze."

She knew lots of men were upfront about their sexuality these days so the fact that this singer wanted to be excused for kissing some other guy didn't seem all that earth-shattering. But Jane went mad. She charged into the bedroom, wild-eyed and grabbed an umbrella from the corner.

Sleepily, Bella asked: "Is George gay then?" as her aunt started to smash the curved end of the brolly up at the ceiling. Bella was still trying to burrow down under the duvet when the umbrella broke and Jane barged into the hall, threw a coat over her nightie and stalked barefoot out of the flat. She was clutching the broken umbrella like a dangerous weapon.

Knock Knock, Who's There?

Upstairs in his circular turret room George was totally oblivious to the protest from below. Even when Jane hurled herself at his door he didn't hear a thing. For one night only George really thought he was the living reincarnation of Jimi Hendrix. All his lights were blazing and he was singing along with the music, strutting round the bedroom before stopping, every so often, to poke his head through the open window and yell: "'Scuse me, while I kiss this guy..." into the sleeping streets below.

Ray was too drunk to bother about the racket and Jane knew Renee was too deaf to care. Jim had been ill for weeks and finally been readmitted to hospital after a TV weather girl told him a tidal wave was about to swamp the West Midlands. Only Amanda and Winston came out of their flats to join Jane in hammering on George's door. None of them were sure where Wendy the warden was.

After they'd collapsed helplessly against the doorway, their ears ringing and too tired to bang any more, Winston said: "Ah well, at least you two can listen to my latest - Knock knock, who's there?"

"Not now Winston!" said Jane and Amanda in perfect unison. Somehow their pent-up frustration was eased. Both had to smile, ruefully, at the house comedian in his woolly Rastafarian hat, no doubt knitted by his mum.

Amanda produced her roll-up cigarette machine and a pouch of tobacco which, Jane guessed, would be mixed with hash. After lighting up,

Amanda offered the spliff to Winston who took a couple of puffs before passing it on to Jane.

Shaking her head, Jane explained: "I'm always frightened of that stuff."

"So am I," said Winston, inhaling deeply. "You know, I reckon it was weed that made me paranoid in the first place. Mum says I'm far too cheerful to be in a place like this – it's only all those folk talking about me that gets on my nerves."

Street-smart Amanda, whose multiple nose and ear piercings had actively helped her land a part-time receptionist's job with an urban-cool advertising agency, became reflective.

"You know, there's no reason why Wendy should always be here. She isn't actually our babysitter."

"And she's not our gaoler either," put in Winston, "but right now we could do with her using that master key she has to get into George's place."

The music was as loud as ever - still Hendrix - still the same song as far as Jane could tell. She wondered whether she should give up and go back to comfort Bella. The child would never get up for school in the morning.

Amanda said: "Now I come to think of it, I was talking to Wendy last week and she said something about her friend's 40th birthday party. I bet that was tonight."

"You were talking to Wendy?" said Jane. "I thought none of us talked to Wendy."

"I've decided she's not so bad – in fact she's not all that different from us," shrugged the one-time secretary turned rough sleeper. Jane and Winston stared at Amanda in amazement.

"Well, you know how I'm always having to wash my hands every five minutes – I rub them raw sometimes. Well, she told me how she was once diagnosed with OCD – you know obsessive compulsive disorder."

"I know what it means," nodded Jane tetchily, wishing she'd brought her own cigarettes upstairs. "Anyway, what was Wendy compulsive about? Sniffing disapprovingly at people?"

The other two thought this was hugely funny although Jane knew she was being mean. Wendy did her best. They got off the floor and after taking turns to give five more bashes on George's door, they all gave up and headed back to their own beds. Each was determined to break every one of George's CDs the next day.

Bella was fast asleep when Jane got back downstairs, her ears hidden under the pillow. Wearily, Jane lit up and made herself comfortable in the lounge. There was nothing to do now but wait for the slugs to put in an appearance. George would have to do one hell of a lot of removal jobs to make up for tonight.

She'd managed to nod off by the time Bella woke up. The music was still on upstairs although the volume was less. As usual the ashtray was overflowing but Bella knew her aunt would be upset if she tried to empty it into the kitchen bin. Jane was meticulous about grinding her cigarettes to a pulp and wouldn't allow any ashtray to be emptied unless it had been standing for at least a day. She was also forever checking the batteries in the smoke alarm after a bathroom curtain incident she preferred not to talk about.

Bella knew it had been a rough night for her aunt and had no intention of waking her up. Instead she opened a new tin of food for Mr C, who was never allowed to leave scraps in his bowl anymore. It hadn't stopped the slugs coming back. They already knew their way through the cat flap and slithered in, hopefully, most nights.

"It's a good job I'm not too squeamish," shuddered Bella, screwing up her face as she tried to shove newspaper under a couple. After dropping the slugs into the empty can of cat meat she checked the lid. It read: "Sorry, you have not won the £1 million bonus this time. Keep Trying."

*****

Bella was into her third week at Peacehaven Mansions when Mary rang to report her mum was very close to coming round and the doctors believed she would make a full recovery. By then another minor miracle had happened. Jane was making more of an effort to cut down on the cigarettes. She spent a lot of time smoking on the doorstep and confined her heaviest sessions to the middle of the night when she pushed open the window facing the brick wall and practically froze to death.

The downside was Jane had taken to sweets and chocolates with a vengeance and was always nipping out to the shops, or begging Bella to go for her. One night, as Bella sat at the kitchen table wrestling with decimals, Jane absently munched through a whole box of Maltesers, offering her niece just one. Catching an accusing glance, as she groped for the last chocolate, Jane didn't apologise. She just said: "You don't want teeth like mine."

Ray's drinking was more of a problem. He could be so thoughtful when he was sober. Drunk, he turned into a foul-mouthed demon nobody recognised. And he wasn't cooking.

Bella knew her grandmother had sent a cheque for extra food. But Jane's efforts to cut down smoking during the day ended up with her waving Bella off to school then collapsing into her still warm bed. There was never any time to get to the bank.

After her first flash of enthusiasm, regular food in the house was becoming increasingly hit and miss. The trouble was Jane was always distracted by her own health problems. Even the reality of a sister lying hundreds of miles away in a hospital bed didn't prevent her from firmly believing that she was the sick one. Sandy would be all right. Sandy had always been all right, she insisted, forgetting once again, to buy any milk.

The hunt for something to spread inside Bella's school sandwiches was a constant source of late night trips to the off-licence. By the end of the third week they'd had baked beans for tea twice, a burnt casserole made in a sober moment by Ray but then left too long in the oven by Jane, and some economy frankfurters. Bella was grateful for invitations to tea at the homes of her two best friends, whose mothers' were astonished by her appetite. These same mothers would often press Bella to stay the night. But the child always wanted to get back to Peacehaven Mansions even though she was probably facing a late-night door knock round the other flats in a bid to borrow butter, sugar, or teabags.

The only breakfast cereal was always cornflakes. Despite Bella's hints and post-it notes, fruit-flavoured yoghurts and muesli - or rabbit food as Jane called it - were never on the menu.

On the plus side, Aunty Jane was never running off to important meetings. She was never running off anywhere except to the newsagent. In the evenings Winston liked coming down to listen to her practising the guitar and afterwards there was usually an old video to watch. If Bella woke in the night, worried about her mum, Jane was always ready to talk. As long as her niece could cope with the smoke, she'd talk without embarrassment about any subject under the sun. Her own life may have been unfulfilled but Jane was boundless in her enthusiasm for Bella's future.

So were all the other tenants of Peacehaven Mansions. As they searched their meagre cupboards to pass on out-of-date cheese spreads or their last slices of bread, each of them wanted to know how Bella was, what she was doing at school, what she wanted to do when she left. Her brief presence in the house had already come to represent a beacon of hope for people like virtually housebound Renee and compulsive hand-washer Amanda. If this child flourished then the world was perhaps not quite such an unfair and chaotic place.

When Bella confessed to having a bit of a thing for one of the boys at school, Jane was eager to know what he was like even though she warned it was important not to let infatuation blind you to the realities of somebody's true personality.

Somehow, Bella knew her aunt was chatting and sharing secrets in the same way she must have chatted to her mum when they were young girls. She missed her mother so much. Often the late night conversations calmed her. Aunty Jane was the next best thing.

Chapter 19

If the hunger pangs really set in, Jane would march up to the Queen's Head and yank Ray back to the house. He already kept all his pans and scary-looking knives in Jane's kitchenette and, despite his obvious inebriation, could always turn out a mouthwatering Spanish omelette.

Jane's deranged appearance in the pub did not go unremarked. The Beddows brothers never missed her dramatic entrances or the instant effect she had on the thin "little tosser" who practically cowered whenever she showed up.

Something had to be done.

On Thursday Amanda suggested Ray took George to the pub with him so the rest of them could have some peace. But George had already spent most of his disability living allowance that month and could only afford a couple of pints. Ray forked out for a couple more but it still meant "Purple Maze," Haze, or whatever, was dominating Bella's homework by 8.30pm.

Next morning, as she stood, sleepily at the bus stop, Renee made one of her rare outside appearances and walked slowly up the road to join Bella. As usual, (delete she'd) Renee had left a note written in careful block capitals pinned to her front door. The message read: "Back Soon, Mum."

The oldest tenant of Peacehaven Mansions seemed even more agitated than   normal about leaving her watching post at the window and kept looking back over her shoulder. Then she confided

that the previous night she'd seen two men
following George down the road from the pub.
Bella wondered if they were his gay friends. As the
bus lumbered into view she decided not to share
the thought with Renee, who might be shocked.
But later that night, after most of them had gone to
bed, the words: "Pervert" and a more wobbly
"Peedofile," were spray-painted on the side of the
house.
On Saturday Wendy was practically hysterical. "I
knew this would happen, I knew it!" she wailed,
waking Jane and Bella up at 7am.
"I've told them at head office this place isn't
suitable for a child. Now look what's happened!
And I'm sorry Jane, but you have taken advantage
of my better nature. First it seems this child was
living here for a week before you bothered to
inform me…then you said it would only be for
another couple of days."
Standing on the doorstep Wendy hardly drew
breath as her voice rose higher and higher. "I
should have pushed social services to get their act
together. If they weren't always on sick leave or
maternity leave or some other leave they'd have
been down here straight away. This child needs
proper supervision – not a home with people
who…who…well, who've all been in a psychiatric
hospital."
As Bella looked round for Mr C, Jane angrily
reminded Wendy that this was supposed to be her
home and as a tenant she could surely have
whoever she wanted visiting. Wendy seemed to
forget that Bella had come to stay because of a

family crisis. The conversation ended with Jane saying through tight lips, that she would "sort something out".

"Yes, well…" sniffed Wendy. "I know things are difficult, I don't mean to sound unreasonable. Perhaps I'd better go and ring the police. There's a real yob element living round here…I just can't be responsible for everything with no direction…"

At that moment Ray blundered blearily out of his flat wearing trainers and his pyjama bottoms. The ribs stuck out in his chest which was practically hairless and stark white.

"Get the fucking coppers," said Ray, peering at the scrawl. "Sorry for the language Bella but someone needs arresting for that. It's slander. I knew those bleeders at the pub were smirking at me when they strolled back in last night – why didn't I see what they'd done when I got back?"

Nobody wanted to point out that Ray hardly saw anything when he blundered back to his flat after closing time at the Queen's Head.

"I know exactly who's responsible," repeated Ray. And if those creeps can afford to buy cans of paint why can't they buy a bloody dictionary!"

Bella found herself holding Mr C in a grip too close for comfort. She wanted her mother.

"What if they come back? When are the police coming?" she asked.

"Don't worry, I'm going to ring them straight away," said Wendy. "And Ray, perhaps you could please stay away from that pub for a few days. Just until our young guest here can…get sorted out."

Knock Knock, Who's There?

Ray was about to reply with more expletives when Jane cut him off. "Come on, Ray, come and watch early-morning cartoons with me and Bella. I'll make you a coffee."

Bella felt a bit guilty leaving Wendy alone in the driveway. She suspected the caretaker might also have wanted to be invited in for a bit of company right then. But what could she do? Her aunt never wanted Wendy "snooping around."

Sighing, Wendy turned and hurried back to her own flat where she bolted the door even though it was still early morning. The telephone at the police station rang out for ages before she was finally put through to the duty sergeant for the area.

After giving brief details, Wendy was told a PC Roberts would call round and take a statement when he came on duty later that day. Putting the phone down she wondered whether she should have rung 999. Ill feeling in the area seemed to be escalating. The situation looked like a potential emergency to her.

Chapter 20

The kitten had been a mistake. Thrashing around sleepless, in her hospital bed, Sandy now realised she had imposed an extra burden on her sister. Even cats needed some attention and Jane needed all her energy just to keep on getting up every morning. Well, perhaps every afternoon would be more accurate.

"Why do I never learn?" murmured Sandy. Through the darkness, her mother's voice answered her.

"Never learn what? How are you feeling love?"

"Why? Where? Mum! Is this a dream?"

Mary's kind face swam into view in a halo of light above the darkened bed.

"Not any more. But it has been a nightmare waiting and waiting for you to properly wake up. Oh Sandra, I've been so worried about you…"

Drops of moisture began to fall from the well-loved face, leaving Sandy more convinced than ever that she'd slipped into some parallel universe. Sandra! Her mother always called her Sandra when she was in trouble.

It was only when the main light was switched on that Sandy dimly remembered she was in a hospital ward. There was a bowl of fruit on the side table and this elderly woman sobbing on a chair. Her mother. It was Mary wearing a black polo neck jumper and a crumpled tweed skirt. I've told her black is all wrong for her skin tones – it's so ageing, reflected Sandy, drifting into PR mode.

Knock Knock, Who's There?

Aloud she said: "Mother, where's that plum-coloured cardigan I bought you last Christmas?" For some reason the question made her mother burst out laughing, and then start crying again. It was weird.

Then Sandy remembered. There was a crash. In the mountains. Roger had been bleeding….what happened to Roger?

"Mum! Where's Roger?"

"Shhush. Safe, he's safe dear... Look, I've rung for the nurse. You have to take it very slowly. You've had a terrible shock."

What terrible shock? Sandy couldn't remember any shock…unless there was something she'd forgotten.

Bella! Where was Bella…"BELLA!" she sat up and screamed. "Where is Bella?"

Nurses in nuns' habits hurried into the room and Sandy grew dizzy and sank back down again. Slowly her mother's soothing words penetrated the fog that had dropped down over the bed like a shroud.

"Bella is absolutely fine," repeated Mary, over and over. "You remember. She's staying with Jane. They're having a good time together. She's learning to cook. Shush, listen. You can talk to Bella on the telephone in a little while when she gets back from school. Shush…shush…."

More than anything Mary wanted to cradle her younger daughter in her arms and sing her to sleep like a baby. Instead, she contented herself with making cooing noises, as if to a child, while the nurses checked Sandy's blood pressure, took

her temperature and nodded to each other.
Before going off to fetch a doctor, one of them
smiled at Mary and said: "Bon! She is return-ed."

*****

Roger hobbled in to see Sandy as soon as the
doctor left. "What's a beautiful woman like you
doing in a place like this?" he asked, grinning
widely.
Sandy felt the tears prickling in the corners of her
eyes as she looked up into his wonderful dark
eyes, half-hidden by a tangle of unruly hair.
"Rog, I'm so sorry about the accident. Your poor
leg. It will mend, won't it?"
"Hey, I've got another one. These things happen.
It was an accident."
"But supposing it had been your hands – that's
how you make your living!"
"Will you stop going on about me – it's you that
gave us all the scare. You've been slipping in and
out of consciousness for nearly three weeks."
"Well not any more. I'm back – but worried stiff
about Bella."
She came here, remember? To see you and you
woke up and spoke to her. Listen, from what I can
gather, she's been okay. She misses you but
she's going to school every day and sounds fine
on the phone. Your mother can tell you more but it
strikes me you underestimate your 'little girl.' You
wait, she'll have Jane jumping off that sofa and
down to the Jobcentre before you can blink. She

just doesn't carry all the emotional baggage you and Jane have between you."

Sandy was unconvinced.

"I'm still worried about her staying in such a tiny flat with no escape from all that smoke. Jane can't give up even if she wanted to, then half the other residents walk in and light up as well. Bella's never had a strong chest."

"Obviously you've never heard her on the clarinet. Not that she's any good, but she's damn loud. Believe me, her lungs were alive and very well when I last heard them in action. Still, she should concentrate on the guitar. And you should concentrate on getting better and back to business. I keep having to field calls from that PA of yours about the progress of some footballer on his charity walk. What do I know about football?"

Sandy relaxed. "I wonder if that doctor is talking to Mum about when they might discharge me?"

"Well, they've told me I can go in a day or two but I don't reckon you'll be going anywhere for another week at least."

Suddenly, Sandy felt wistful. "Of course, you're right, Bella is better with Jane than I am. She makes her laugh and they play Scrabble and Monopoly together for hours."

Then she was weeping. "Why don't I make my sister laugh, Roger? I try so hard to help her but it all seems for nothing. One day she's back, my sister, just as she always was. And we're so close. Next day she's slipped back into that bottomless pit of depression and I just can't get in and reach her. D'you understand? I win her back only to lose her all over again. Somehow that's more hurtful than if she'd never been back at all…no, no, I don't mean that…"

As Sandy's distress mounted, Roger hobbled round the bed to put his arms around her. "I know, I know. Listen gorgeous, when someone's really good at what they do for a living , like you are, it can make other people, like your big sister – like me for God's sake – sometimes feel a bit of a failure. I mean you're so successful running that business, and she's sort of thrown her life away…"

As Sandy began to protest, Roger rushed on: "All right, all right, not thrown it away – she's been unlucky. But that's not your fault so why feel so guilty? Everybody has good times and bad times. Right now we haven't had the best of luck either…."

Sandy flopped back onto the pillows and gazed up at the man she now knew she wanted to wake up with every morning. Her head began to ache. How can he say we're not lucky, she thought, fighting to keep her eyes open.

Chapter 21

Brian Beddows did own a dictionary and could have spelt paedophile. But it was not him, it was his dyslexic brother Ian who'd been responsible for the graffiti at Fruitcake Towers. Ian had arrived back at the pub, flushed with success, accompanied by some kid with spiked hair who he slapped on the back and offered to buy a drink. As usual Ray was there, but for once, both brothers tried hard not to look in his direction.

"Sup up Ian, I'll get you another," growled Brian, who had been doing some thinking. "You know, if we can get rid of the alcoholic 'perv,' the rest of that effing shower would follow. You'll see."

Tapping the side of his nose, Brian told Ian it might not be a bad idea to investigate where they could both get loans. After all, the old house might end up back on the market and was sure to go for some knock-down price. If they could only get their hands on a bit of capital they might be able to buy it and rent it to students. Better still, "young professionals."

Two days later, after the brothers had taken their wives to see Bruce Willis in Diehard 4, they'd called in at the Queen's Head on the way home. There was no way either man could relax once they found the "little perv" propping up their bar, yet again. Just after 11pm they watched as Ray half-fell off his stool, then staggered out.

Something inside Brian snapped. Enough was enough.

"Got a bit of business to do, love," Brian said to his wife, Julie. "Here's a fiver, you and Gemma get yourselves a taxi home, we'll be back soon." Ignoring the protests from both women, the brothers began looking round for allies. Brian approached one-time school bully Brett Ansley, who was carrying too much weight these days but had always been handy with his fists. While he was outlining the dire situation down the road, the old Peacehaven gardener, Ken, must have overheard because he got up from a nearby table and muttered: "I'm with you."

"Naw grandad, have another pint on me, believe me this is not something you want to get involved with," said Brian.

But the stubborn old bugger put on his overcoat and said: "I know the grounds of that place like the back of my hand - I can be useful. " Thumping his fist into his other hand, Ken Cracknell added, meaningfully: "And what you don't know is I used to be a miner before I went into 'orticulture."

Jesus, the last thing Brian wanted was some geriatric hanging around. Still, if they got down the road fast enough the poor devil wouldn't be able to keep up. Saturday was a good night for a ruck. All the coppers would be down town dealing with young hooligans.

"Okay grandad – Ken, isn't it? Well, Brett's going first with his mobile phone, then me and our Ian will follow. You can be our rear guard, so give us five minutes. Right?"

Brian and Ian were halfway down the road when Brett phoned back to report: "The little tosser was

staggering about all over the place but that chain-smoking bint's just dragged him in to 'er place."
Jane was having a cigarette at the door as Ray, who was born in Leeds, stumbled up the drive singing "Maybe it's because I'm a Londoner..."
She smiled and called out: "Ray, come in for a coffee. Bella's watching one of those Terminator films on my video. I've been avoiding that scene in the mental hospital; it should be over by now."
As soon as he veered into Jane's flat, Ray switched on to auto-pilot, tied on an old striped apron and slapped the frying pan on the stove. He was sizzling sausages and singing at the top of his voice when there was a bang on the door and the sound of milk bottles being smashed.
Jane and Bella jumped but Ray carried on frying and singing, oblivious to the noise. Jane crept to the front door and peered through her security spy-hole. A great bruiser of a man she didn't know was outside.
"What do you want?"
"Bit of a chat with our mutual acquaintance," snarled Brett. "Have you got a kid in there – schoolgirl, about eleven?"
"What's that got to do with you?"
Suddenly Brian loomed into view, banging louder and kicking violently at the door. Jane recognised him from the pub. His nose looked huge against the magnifying spy hole. She could see his blackheads.
From somewhere on the darkened drive Jane heard another lout yelling. As the noise outside

grew louder, Ray stopped singing and carefully switched off the gas.

Through the letterbox Jane shouted: "I'm getting the police." Bella began to whimper as Ray flung down a tea towel and lurched towards the door, mouthing obscenities. Jane's heart was pounding as she tried to take control of the situation. She said: "Bella, ring 999....Ray, listen to me, you're not going out there...you're not going out there..." As Ray tried to push Jane aside, the sound of their arguing and Bella crying, spurred Brian and his gang to kick even harder at the door. Something heavy, a plant pot, or a brick, was thrown.

A voice bawled: "Get out here you dirty pervert....get out and clear out...we don't want your type round here!"

"What type is that then," yelled Ray, who against all his better instincts, and years of experience in the hotel trade, finally broke free of Jane and wrenched open the front door.

Desperately, Jane tried to hang on to the strings of his apron as Ray charged out, incandescent with rage, and started swinging his emaciated fists in all directions. Brian was on him like a flash. Even though one of Ray's wild punches actually connected with somebody's jaw he was thumped in the stomach and bent double.

There were three of them circling him, as he groaned, each of them dabbing out, kicking, urging the other to get stuck in, then holding back, as if steeling themselves before going in for the kill.

Knock Knock, Who's There?

Still trying to hold on to Ray, Jane was swung round and fell down, scraping her knees. She looked up to see Bella's terrified face in the doorway, her hand clinging onto the cordless phone. From the ground Jane screamed: "Don't you dare come out here, slam that door get the police."

But the child's first instinct was to drop the phone and rush out to help.

"No, no! Get back! Lock the door," pleaded Jane, staggering back to her feet.

Confused, Bella ran back into the house and picked up the frying pan of sausages. As soon as she appeared back in the doorway Jane snatched the pan and bashed Brian over the head. He hardly flinched.

There had to be something heavier...no sharper...a knife. Shoving Bella back towards the door, Jane darted into the flat and grabbed Ray's roll of chef's knives. But the first things that fell out were a barbecue fork and a kebab skewer. They would have to do.

Upstairs, Winston had woken up, got out of bed and was peering down from the fire escape trying to work out what was happening. He couldn't find his glasses and it was difficult to see in the narrow shaft of light coming from Jane's doorway. Bewildered, Winston was wondering whether to go down and investigate when he was elbowed out of the way by Amanda, swearing and shrieking as she ran past, jumped on the fire escape ladder to make it drop, then clanged down the metal stairs in her high heels clutching an aerosol can. Once

on the ground the three thugs brushed off
Amanda's kung-fu style chops but her spray can
of Mace made all three back off for a minute.
Jane, back outside with her meat skewer in one
hand and the barbecue fork in the other, was
frightened of stabbing into the indistinguishable
brawling backs. Instead she went for the soft
option. Bottoms.
First she jabbed the sharp prong into what turned
out to be Ian's backside and saw him leap up in
pain.
"Ow! Get off me you bleeding old witch," he
whined.
Next she plunged the fork into the biggest
backside on view. God, this lout had to be 20
stone pinning down little Ray - the rotten coward.
Meanwhile Brian had already caught an earful of
Mace from Amanda who he'd pushed over just as
Jane caught him in the left buttock with the
skewer.
Brett, undeterred by his own puncture wounds,
had got Ray by the scruff of the neck and was
kicking out with his steel-toed boots when all of a
sudden, he let go, with a yelp. Jane fervently
hoped Ray's foot had caught the fat thug in the
groin. But it was water, pouring down from above.
Boiling water. A whole kettleful splashing red hot
drops onto the gang below.
"Bloody 'ell, Renee, watch where you're pouring
that damn water," yelled Ray, looking up and
twisting away from one of Brett's boots in the nick
of time.

Knock Knock, Who's There?

"You'd better all clear off, I've just put the kettle on to boil again," shouted Renee. "Stay out of my line of fire Ray!"

"Quick," said Jane. "Go and put our kettle on Bella. Go on, move! And ring 999!"

"Shall I put some coffee on then?" called Winston from the floor above. He was still feeling confused.

Ken Cracknell arrived, out of breath, just as Wendy began flapping up and down the drive, running backwards and forwards from her flat screaming: "Ray, Ray, I've rung the police, I've rung the police..."

Ken slipped in behind an overgrown pyracantha bush and watched with disgust as the mad smoking woman used some sort of blades to threaten the men from the pub. Somebody in a room upstairs was trying to burn them with hot water. At least it looked like the drunk lying on the floor had been given a good seeing to. Didn't look like he'd be shooting his mouth off again any time soon.

Finally, manic George was roused by the racket. He emerged from his bedroom turret demanding to know what all the commotion was about. Despite his tattoos, George wasn't really a hard man. He began to shake violently when he saw Ray on the ground, bleeding.

"G-g-g-ot to do something, g-g-got to do something...get help," spluttered George. Where was everybody? Suddenly he turned and raced back to his room with an idea.

*****

Afterwards, the thing most neighbours remembered about the midnight seige of Fruitcake Towers was being jolted awake by the sound of Pink Floyd's 'Astronomy Domine" being belted out at ear-shattering decibels. One or two even recognised it as the opening track on the band's 1967 album, Piper At The Gates Of Dawn.

The whine of police sirens was already adding a high octave top note to the psychedelic backbeat as Jane backed towards her door, still waving a bloodied skewer in one hand and a fork in the other. Cursing, and already scalded from Renee's kettle, overweight, middle-aged bully boy Brett lumbered off into the night.

But none of the dressing gown-clad crowd gathered outside the big house that night was in any doubt it had been Jane, wild-eyed and wielding her barbecue implements, who had really tackled the drunken louts. She'd been ably-assisted by street-fighting secretary Amanda, who'd been hit on the nose and her Mace can sent flying. Brian, snarling, red-faced, burned and dripping with sweat, was holding on to his bleeding backside as two policemen raced up the drive, grabbed the weapons....and arrested Jane.

"No, no...you've got the wrong person," spluttered Wendy, who had been waiting at the end of the drive to wave the patrol car in. During the confusion elderly Ken melted away into the darkness.

Ian was also doing his best to sink into the shadows when a second police patrol car arrived and he was grabbed and handcuffed.

"We were only trying to talk to this bugger – just look what him and the rest of this effing madhouse has done to us," shouted Brian, clutching his bottom. Fortunately, Ray's swollen face and ripped apron, as he groaned on the ground, convinced the policemen of the type of conversation they'd been having.

An ambulance was called and Ray was given first aid at the scene then taken to hospital with suspected broken ribs. Brian and Ian kept saying loudly that they needed to go to hospital too, but refused to lower their trousers when the paramedic asked to examine their injuries.

In the end both brothers were also placed under arrest and Brett was picked up on the road, one hand on his punctured bottom, the other on his scalded cheek. Despite her protestations of self-defence, Jane remained under arrest and was asked to go back to the station for further questioning.

After Jane kicked up a fuss, Bella was allowed to accompany her aunt. Still shaking with fear, part of the child couldn't help feeling thrilled by the prospect of a late-night ride in the back of a police car. It was only after the officers had taken statements from most of the other tenants and talked at length to Wendy, that Jane and Bella were given a lift back home. Jane was warned she was on police bail and might be formally charged in the morning.   Renee used her boiling kettle to make tea.

*****

Next day the first edition of the Evening Echo did nobody at Peacehaven Mansions any favours.
"FORMER PATIENTS IN STABBING CLASH WITH NEIGHBOURS..." screamed the banner headline. After that was a smaller sub-heading reading: "KEBABBED - NO PEACE AT THE HAVEN."
The report that followed said four people had been arrested during a brawl at a half-way house for former mental patients in Cranmere. It was not clear what had started the fight but police agreed that kettles of boiling water, pepper spray and barbecue utensils had been used. As a result one man was now in hospital and three others had been treated for burns and stab wounds and later allowed home.
Some neighbours told reporters they thought the fight had resulted from a party that had got out of hand with loud music, drink and drugs. Others agreed that 'noisy gatherings' were a familiar feature of life at Peacehaven Mansions. Still fuzzy about what had gone on, Winston read the paper and asked George, Renee and Amanda whether they'd ever been invited to these wild parties he must have slept through.
Wendy, incoherent with rage, demanded to speak to the paper's editor, Jack Grady. He told her in

no uncertain terms that it wasn't the reporter's job to attribute blame when arrests had been made and a court case was pending. All they could do was report the facts.

"The facts. Ha!" said Ray, the next morning when Jane and Bella visited him in hospital with a bunch of grapes.

Chapter 22

Once she was sitting up in bed, Sandy began worrying about everything. Even though she knew nothing about the brawl at Peacehaven Mansions, she understood Bella staying in Jane's flat would create problems – the air was so thick with fumes they'd put the smoke alarm in the bathroom.

Both Mary and Roger did their best to reassure her but Sandy would not be comforted. Mary explained how she'd repeatedly suggested Jane take the child and   temporarily move into Sandy's house. Jane said she couldn't do that because Sandy would only complain about her filling the rooms with smoke. On top of that the house was too big and the neighbours too nosy – always asking her how she was and what she was doing for a living these days.

In desperation Sandy passed on the message that perhaps Roger could stay there with them both. Jane's immediate response was: "I'm not living with Roger."

Mary herself had felt soothed by the continuing daily bulletins between Cranmere and Pau during which Bella told her there was nothing to worry about and how Aunty Jane always tried to smoke at the front door. The child said absolutely nothing about her late-night ride in a police car. Or how she was about to go and visit Ray, who'd been so badly beaten up he was in hospital. Mary seemed to take it for granted that Ray was responsible for most of the catering arrangements. She kept asking anxiously how "the three of them" were getting on.

"Grandma, we're fine," Bella repeated, holding the cordless phone and peering hopefully into the fridge to see if there were any eggs.

When Jane got on the phone – and after all the usual rigmarole about how everybody was – Mary told her Roger had been discharged and was due to board a plane for Britain. One of his friends was going to pick him up. Apparently he'd offered to call round, collect their things and take them both up to Sandy's house before being dropped off at his own place. Roger said he was also prepared to sleep in the spare room if Jane needed some "moral support". Whatever that meant.

After putting the phone down, Jane reminded Bella that she could still go and stay with one of her classmates, or one of her mother's friends. After all it wasn't that long until the end of term.

"You're my friends, I like it here," said Bella, wondering whether Winston had any butter.

Jane said gently: "The trouble is Wendy's really making waves about you being here. We need to sort something out. What's more you'll go mad like the rest of us if you stay here much longer." Then, hardly missing a beat, she added: "Not that there's really anything wrong mentally with me. Apart from a bit of depression. And who wouldn't be depressed if they had my heart condition - all that stuff last night has only added to the strain."

Bella had understood instinctively, and from the age of five, how querying the logic of Aunty Jane's dodgy heart could lead to a rapid transformation from laughter to an all-guns-blazing situation. She could still hear her mother screaming: "We'd all get sodding palpitations if we smoked 60 a day and ate pickled onions before going to bed! There's nothing wrong with your heart – what will it take to convince you?"

Bella, the future diplomat, said quietly: "Aunty Jane, perhaps you ought to have a lie down in the bedroom."

"Perhaps I should," said Jane. "That's very thoughtful of you Bella – you've got so much more sense than most people. I'll only be a couple of hours."

Jane pulled on a nightie and a jumper and vanished into the bedroom. As it turned out for the rest of the night. By the time News At Ten was on and there was still nothing but gentle snoring coming from the bedroom, Bella pulled out her aunt's tobacco-pungent duvet and snuggled down on the settee. Soon she was asleep as the ITV news droned on about the situation in Afghanistan, and was followed by Marlon Brando's Seventies sex film, Last Tango In Paris.

*****

Her mother and Sandy had both said it again.
"How are you?"
Why did everyone always have to ask how you were? thought Jane as she flopped into bed.

Knock Knock, Who's There?

It was the first thing Wendy said as soon as she saw any of the tenants - always: "Hello, how are you?"

She never seemed to realise how it drove everyone mad. Or madder.

Her mother should have known better. But no, as soon as she got on the phone it was always: "How are you Jane? And how's Winston? Ray? Renee?" On and on. They were not well. None of them were. Wasn't that obvious from their present living arrangements?

Sandy was the most regular offender. But woe betide you if you actually tried to tell her how you really were. How many times had Jane tried to explain to them that a simple: "Hello, good to see you," was all that was necessary as a greeting. Of course, Sandy brushed this aside and asked what on earth Jane meant....everybody, everywhere in the country spent their days asking others how they were. That didn't mean they wanted a blow-by-blow account of every cough, spit, hospital appointment or nervous breakdown they'd had in the last 12 months.

"Well, to us it means something different," Jane was forever snapping back.

"How are you?" was what the doctors always asked when they were judging whether to raise, or lower, levels of medication. It was what nurses and social workers said, armed with clipboards and notebooks. And how you were varied, dramatically, from day to day, even minute to minute. It was a question that always required careful consideration. The answer might be information you didn't necessarily want to give away on the grounds that it might be used against you later in evidence.

Talking of evidence, what more was she going to say to the police about her extreme actions during the attack on the house? Of course, they'd wanted to know how she was as well. People on the outside of mental illness just didn't get it. What was wrong with a simple hello?

Chapter 23

"I detest hospitals," said Jane, with venom, after she and Bella had visited Ray and were waiting for the number 32 bus back to Peacehaven Mansions.

He had a lot of bruising and several broken ribs. The doctors said they would keep him in a day or two for observation.

"At least it wasn't the other wing," put in Bella, tentatively.

"Don't pussyfoot around," said Jane, drawing hard on her cigarette. "You mean the loony bin which I know so well. And you're right. The whole atmosphere's completely different. God, I'm cold."

"What was it like when you were in there? I remember coming with Grandma and Grandad when I was little but Mum never really liked me to visit with her. She said it was too upsetting."

"For once I agree with your mum. At one stage they said I was doing cartwheels round the ward while they messed about trying to find the right mix of medication to give me."

"Mmm, I remember an old lady screaming a lot. But that wasn't you," said Bella. Jane finished her cigarette.

"Well, perhaps not that time. 'Course the doctors can be as eccentric as they like - and usually are. I caught one of the younger ones whizzing down the corridor on a skateboard some patient from geriatrics had given him!"

"No! You're making it up," giggled Bella.

Jane laughed herself at the memory. "Oh no I'm not - she told him it would help him do his rounds faster. He agreed – at least until the matron caught him!"

Then Jane shivered, half with cold and half with other reminiscences she'd rather not think about. "It was pretty bad, Bella. Not somewhere you ever want to go, believe me. Mostly they trap you into being a voluntary patient and pretend you can leave at any time. But you can't.

"So you just sort of give up and allow yourself to be looked after by people with bad grammar and emotional problems of their own. You've seen Big Brother? Well, looking back it reminds me of that with the doctors calling us into the diary room one by one.

"At least the nurses got to go home at night. Although I suppose they were just as trapped as we were because even if they were bored, or scared of us, they still needed the money. A lot of them were single parents and divorcees. We used to end up giving them advice about their love lives! The idea of being faithful was completely alien to most of the young ones.

"Personally I liked the Irish nurses best. I always ended up telling them which of the young doctors was worth a second glance. As if I knew anything about men! Anyway, after a bit it was the other patients who probably helped me more than the nurses and doctors."

Jane paused, then added: "Even though it's heart disease that's my real problem."

Knock Knock, Who's There?

Bella took a calculated risk before saying: "Aunty Jane, you don't know for certain it's your heart. Mum says…"

"Never mind what your Mum says," said Jane, widening her eyes and arching both eyebrows. "She doesn't know everything – she's just cultivated an air of knowing everything because of that business of hers stuffed with pampered actors and footballers who hardly know how to wipe their own noses…"

Catching sight of her niece's solemn face, Jane softened.

"No, I don't mean that. She's clever your Mum. Really clever, and brave. That's why she's going to get back on her feet in no time. You'll see."

*****

The Beddows brothers and Brett Ansley were all charged with assault occasioning grievous bodily harm. Their solicitor warned them they could be looking at a prison stretch. Ian had no previous convictions and Brian only one for common assault at a football match years ago. Brett kept his mouth shut. It was always possible the magistrates could pass his case on to the Crown Court, added the solicitor.

Jane, who had fought off their attack with sharp-bladed instruments, was very nearly charged with the same offence. But her arguments about self-defence were accepted and some sort of deal was done with the investigating officer. Instead Jane was asked to go back to the police station where she was formally cautioned about her indiscriminate use of an offensive weapon, namely a barbecue fork.

At their preliminary court hearing, all three men denied the charges and were allowed out on bail on condition that none of them went within 100 metres of Peacehaven Mansions.

But the chairwoman of the bench had not thought to deny then access to their power base at the Queen's Head. For the two nights Ray was in hospital, and then convalescing with a can in his flat, the brothers spread their version of "the truth" about what really happened on the night of the alleged assault.

Even those who doubted some of the details of Brian and Ian's story couldn't escape noticing that neither brother was sitting very comfortably these days. Ian had been off work with a 'back' injury and Brian could never finish a hand of poker - he had to stand up after a while to relieve the pain in his buttocks.

"Bastards!" he winced, to nobody in particular. Their lawyer - who was costing an arm and a leg – suggested they try to come up with a few character witnesses before the trial, which was unlikely to take place for months. Brian nearly had a fit when he found out that Ray, the pervert, would qualify for Legal Aid if he needed it. So would the vicious cow who'd stabbed him.

Knock Knock, Who's There?

"That's just typical of this bleeding country these days!" he stormed. "Penalise the working man but bend over backwards for the ruddy criminal."
A few mates organised a whip round and one of them suggested a charity pool tournament, though it never took place. Ian came up with two old ladies whose guttering he'd cleared. Both were prepared to go to court and speak up for him and his brother. Someone booked the room above the Co-op for another protest meeting about the dangerous loonies living in Fruitcake Towers.

*****

Ray wasn't in hospital long but his absence altered the afternoon routine at the house. Renee, The Watcher, devised a new way of waking Jane up as soon as she saw Bella getting off the bus from school. Instead of banging on her bathroom ceiling to rouse Ray down below, she now thumped sideways to alert George who immediately gave two amplified bursts of whatever was playing on his stereo. As it happened, Jane was awake anyway.
As soon as Bella's key turned in the lock, she was waiting - oven glove at the ready - to put the Good Morning programme's dish of the day on the table. On Monday it was lentil and cauliflower bake with some leftover lamb.
"Lovely," crunched Bella.
In fact, Jane had rung Ray up in hospital to ask how long to soak the lentils. He'd told her overnight but there wasn't time for that. Bella

thought her aunt had more energy than she'd ever seen before and seemed to be oozing with culinary confidence and the motivation to try new things. She kept smiling as she swallowed a lump of possible gristle.

*****

After tea, Bella rang her mother and the pair were able to have their first normal conversation since the accident. Except Sandy went on and on wanting to know how she was coping with the smoke levels in the flat and reminding her to empty all the ashtrays into the dustbin before going to bed.
"You never know with cigarettes," said Sandy.
"Mum, I've been here for weeks…I'm fine," laughed Bella. "Aunty Jane made me this fantastic casserole tonight…here she is, waiting to have a word…"
Bella passed the phone to a nervous looking Jane, whose light tone of a few minutes earlier instantly changed to pure tension.
"I'm glad you're feeling better Sandy…when are you coming back?"
Sadly, Bella followed the stilted conversation between the two people she loved so much. She wanted to cry. Why couldn't her aunt relax?
But when she got back on the phone for a final word with her mother, she realised that it was not only Aunty Jane who was tense.

Knock Knock, Who's There?

"Yes Mum, I'm doing my homework....yes, I've got the laptop...we've been back to our house and the neighbours have watered all the plants and are closing the curtains every night.
"What? Yes, yes, they're opening them up again in the morning! When do the doctors think you can come home?"

Chapter 24

Why couldn't she share a house with Roger?
Jane still did most of her serious sleeping during
the day but when Bella kindly offered her the
chance of an early evening rest in her own room, it
was such a relief to close the bedroom door and
think her own thoughts.
Jane knew she was being unfair and probably
irrational about her sister's boyfriend. There was
no denying it would be good for the child to get
back to her own home. And Bella could hardly go
alone, without some sort of chaperone. What was
it about Roger that put her on guard? Was he
really dodgy or was it just deep-rooted
resentments of her own resurfacing about men? It
wasn't as if she didn't trust Ray, or Winston, or
even George when he was in the right frame of
mind.
Was it just that Roger was her sister's lover? Was
this all just an echo of her bitterness about Bruce,
and his betrayal?

*****

There had been 181 steps up to the parapet
holding the medieval church spire. Jane
remembered counting them, at first silently, then
with mounting hysteria as she snivelled, and
sobbed her way to the top.

Knock Knock, Who's There?

An attendant at the entrance downstairs was chatting to an American tourist. She barely noticed the serious young woman in the summer dress. Except to register the fact that unlike some of the more elderly visitors, this one, at least, looked capable of tackling the spiral staircase. Even though she was back living at home, Jane still had her students' union card so was able to pay the discount admission price of £1.25. The woman assured her that the view from the top was worth the climb.

"There's nobody else up there right now so you won't have any trouble," she said turning back to her only other customer and explaining: "It can get tricky at busy times when somebody coming down has to flatten themselves against the walls to let those going up get past."

"Three, four, five, six…." said Jane under her breath as she began to climb.

She could still hear the attendant's conversation right up to step 32 when her voice finally faded away and Jane suddenly felt very alone.

That was when the other voices, the ones in her head, began to grow louder. Particularly the hateful girl with the singsong voice who seemed to have taken up permanent residence.

"You're doing the right thing….you're doing the right thing…the only thing to do…the only thing to do…." she sang. *"After all, you're just a nuisance…and noooobody loves you….."*

33, 34, 35, 36….

A man's voice broke in. *"Bruce loves her. The boffin said he was leaving his wife…"*

"Bruce doesn't love her….nobody loves Jane…." said the singsong girl. *"Come on, up you go: 37, 38, 39…."*

Jane began panting for breath. Her heart was thumping like a thing possessed. No wonder those doctors had tried to hide their despair when they examined her. She was going to do this. It was quicker, cleaner than a lingering death with tubes and monitors, never knowing when you were going to breathe your last….only knowing it was coming….

"41,42,43,44…." Wait - had she missed one? Better go back. "42,43,44…." What was she doing, for Christ's sake, checking her maths! *"You've been a stupid, gullible little fool…."* said the girl in her head.

"But I still love him…." Jane heard herself sob.

"Well, he doesn't love you….and he has a wife and two adorable pet dogs….Did you forget the springer spaniels Jane? Did you forget them? Did you, did you, did you…?"

The man cut in: *"Come on, she didn't know about the pets. That bastard said nothing about having animals…they were his wife's."*

Jane began to whimper, only softly, but the moans reverberated round the walls, which seemed to be closing in.

" 61, 62, 63, 64…" he said he was going to leave his wife….he, he promised….

"76,77,78,79…." It wasn't just me, but I knew, I knew he had a wife….

"Yes, you knew he had a wife." This time the male and female voice combined and repeated the

words. Jane tried to block them out by covering her ears.

The tears were hot on her cheeks and her nose began to run. She crumpled on a bend and stayed there, breathing hard, searching her coat pocket for a tissue, something, but there was nothing. Bruce. He'd unlocked the whole world for her. Presented life on a plate: success, failure, confidence, working class short-term rewards, middle-class deferred gratification....Deferred gratification for God's sake! Not something he'd practised much himself...not according to that wife of his.

Jane had always liked a good row. She'd enjoyed taking Bruce on in the lecture hall, challenging some of his left-wing bias – or had she been too right-wing? What did it matter...97, 98, 99, 100. He said he enjoyed their clashes, showed somebody out there was listening. Sometimes he made a point of making preposterous comments just to check if they weren't all asleep or hungover from the night before.

Bruce said Jane was far too black and white in her views – she'd worked hard and got into higher education and believed most others could do the same. She'd told him she knew perfectly well there were far brighter   girls at her old school who never wanted to leave the place they knew – it wasn't simply a lack of confidence, or ambition. It was some primeval desire to stay rooted in one place...what was wrong with that?

Bruce smiled and invited her to join him at a fringe socialist group he belonged to – was it Militant?

She couldn't remember. They all seemed very angry and worked up about the class system so perhaps it was....130, 131, 132....

It was the Get Well card he sent that had really upset her. Just Best Wishes, Bruce.

How could he? After all they'd been to each other....

"You mean all you thought you'd been to each other," put in the girl.

...141, 142, 143...I can't go back to Mum and Dad. And Sandy should be in the sixth form by now....I'm holding her back. This mad obsession is blocking everything....I can't go back and live there like a child...I'm twenty and they can't help me, they can't help me....they've tried but they just can't help me...159, 160, 161, 162...

Jane's breath was coming in ever-shorter bursts. It was the heart, of course. From now on everything would always be a strain on her faulty heart valves....She had to stop because she could hardly see for the tears.

The hem of her dress was the only remedy for her streaming nose....who cared...who'd ever know now....To drown out the voices Jane began speaking aloud: "Mother, I'm sorry....I'm so sorry but you can't help me and Dad can't help me and Sandy can't see why I can't get myself together. Anyway, she's got her whole life ahead of her...My illness is going to ruin everything for her. Oh God help me, help me...make it quick, please make it quick...."

...178, 179, 180...*"One hundred and eighty"* boomed the man's voice in darts match triumph.

Knock Knock, Who's There?

Finally, she was at the top and it was so cold. The parapet had castellated edges and you could see the whole city bathed in golden late afternoon sunlight. A flock of pigeons flew by, then a fat, lone one fluttered up from below and perched, unsteadily, on the edge of the stonework. One of its feet was an ugly, clawed ball.

When Jane looked over the parapet edge she saw the top of a gargoyle covered in white droppings. The pigeon cooed then flew off, gliding downwards on some thermal.

"This is it," said the girl and man simultaneously. *"Jump, jump, jump...."*

Jane put one leg onto the lowest part of the stonework and gripped the top of the parapet with the other hand. People down below looked like dots. Her heart was hammering and for a minute she gazed up at a plane, passing overheard. Why couldn't she be heading for Spain with a party of holidaymakers?

"Wheeee, she's going to do it," giggled the girl.

 "Please don't do this," said the man's voice.

No. It wasn't the same man. It was another, gentler voice.

Jane's breathing was so loud that she didn't, at first, distinguish the different accent. A quick glance over her shoulder showed there was someone standing behind her.

"Go away, s-s-stay back," she stammered.

But the voice coming from the stranger's mouth carried on speaking. It dawned on Jane this had to be the American she'd seen at the entrance to the tower. It seemed he was more than a tourist. He had a dog collar round his neck and was saying something about coming to serve in England for a few months...serve what? What was he talking about?

"Go away, leave me alone, I've g-g-got to do this," she'd repeated.

"No, no, you don't" said the man, blinking furiously as he took a step closer.

"Of course, you do," said the sing-song girl. *"Now jump, jump, jump...."*

But the spell was broken. So was her nerve. With infinite patience, the trainee priest had reached out his hand and just held it there ...until Jane found her fingers clasping his.

"Shall we go and get some coffee," he drawled. "Or would a nice English girl like you prefer tea?"

The woman at the bottom of the tower had given them a funny look as they walked out together, the curate and the young girl.

He's a fast worker, she thought to herself.

Round the corner they found a chintzy teashop where the American had insisted on having strong black coffee with a toasted teacake. Jane's hands shook as she held the bone china teacup to her lips.

She told him all about Bruce and how she couldn't get him out of her head.

"I have no solutions for love, and I'm sure no expert," said the curate. "All I can suggest is you give things just a little more time."

"You mean, because he might come back?" asked Jane, hating the eagerness in her tone.

Knock Knock, Who's There?

"I mean because you need to give yourself time to come to terms with how things are," said the man of God, who'd taken her home in a taxi, insisting on paying the fare. He'd spoken for a few minutes to her mum and dad and promised to come round and see her again.

But when he did, Jane was already in hospital.

Chapter 25

"There always seems to be somebody watching the house these days," Renee told Jane. She'd telephoned downstairs from her upstairs look-out point.

As usual Jane had dragged herself from sleep and stayed awake long enough to see Bella off to school. But although Jane's 'lights were on,' as Ray liked to say, 'there was nobody really at home.'

Jane kissed Bella goodbye, pressed some jam sandwiches and a badly bruised apple into her bag, and tried to concentrate on what Renee was saying.

"I don't know who it is but I catch glimpses. At night I can just feel someone out there," said Renee. "I've told Wendy but she thinks I'm imagining things." Wedging the phone under her ear Jane leaned out of the front door, pulling the edges of her dressing gown over her chest. She couldn't really see anything from that angle but decided to show some solidarity. What else did Renee have to do but look out of her window all day. And she wasn't usually paranoid.

"Could it be that lot from the Queen's Head again?" asked Jane, going cold.

"I don't think so. I've seen that big red-faced man with the sore arse – you know the one I scalded a few times – but only in the distance. And there's a real tarty-looking woman with spiky high heels who always tuts when she passes by. She might be from the pub. But I don't think it's them watching us. It's somebody else."

"Sure you're not having a funny turn, Renee?" asked Jane, lighting up and cringing, as she waited for a burst of outrage down the line. When there was only silence, she added: "And Wendy hasn't noticed anyone?"

"Wendy's too worried about this protest meeting they're having tonight at the Co-op. Well, in the dance hall over the Co-op – I remember it had a lovely sprung floor…"

"Oh come on, nobody'll go to that," said Jane scornfully. "It's half past seven, Coronation Street's on."

"Wendy's asked me and Winston if we'll say a few words – fat chance, as far as I'm concerned."

"The council put us in here, let them say a few words," said Jane. "What else do we pay our taxes for?"

"D'you pay tax?" asked Renee, incredulously.

"Course not, but you know what I mean," said Jane.

*****

"Right then, most of you know me - Frank Marshall, chairman of the Cranmere Tenants' and Residents' Association - and this is Bill Howarth from social services. We've called this meeting following several complaints coming from this area about Peacehaven Mansions – the house up the road for ex-ment…I mean, recovering psychiatric patients.

"Joining us on the platform is Councillor Burberry, who represents this area for Labour and Cllr Minshell, who'll be standing as an Independent in the local elections in May."

"Get on with it…." yelled a man in the audience.

"Let me say at the outset, I'll tolerate no interruptions of that kind. You'll all get your chance to speak," said Frank, who ran his own building company and was used to handling awkward customers.

"Not if you don't shut up we won't…."

Frank stiffened but decided to ignore the heckling. He'd got a cousin with clinical depression and felt he had a better grasp on the problems of mental health than most. Not that he had much time for Uncle Bill's lad, but that was another story. None of the local residents had wanted Peacehaven Mansions to be converted into a place for ex-nutters. As chairman of the association Frank had been asked to raise formal objections with the council. But that didn't mean he was totally insensitive. Just thinking about his own kids, and the young apprentices at work, Frank did understand how easy it was to lose your grip when you were just starting out in life. The wrong job, a girlfriend ditching you, bad A levels in a record-breaking year - it didn't take much to knock a person off- balance.

Councillor Burberry had helped him put out extra chairs after nearly   50 people turned up to voice their concerns following the "stabbing incident". It was clear many were worried and a few downright angry, particularly a bunch of belligerent rowdies at the back.

Most just wanted to know what had happened on the night of the assaults. Perhaps this oddball Winston could throw some light on the subject, thought Frank. Pity he was black – might not help the prejudiced among them. The harmless-looking old woman hadn't shown up. He could see Wendy, the caretaker, sitting in the corner. Instinctively, Frank knew she might be more of a hindrance than a help and was likely to come over as some middle-class do-gooder. Dick Burberry already looked out of his depth. He'd taken over the safe Labour seat less than a year ago and had probably never faced so many hostile voters in the same room before. A man in the front row got things under way.

He said: "My wife's worried to death since you moved that loony lot into the old house. What the hell was anyone thinking about having them right in the middle of a residential area? It's less than a quarter of a mile from a primary school!"

"What about the incident with the knife?" demanded a Sikh in a turban.

Frank wondered whether he was carrying his ceremonial sword. Dynamic young social services deputy director Bill Howarth, who wore an earring and always looked half-cut to Frank, suddenly jerked up his head and snapped: "The so-called incident with the blade – I think you'll find it was a barbecue implement - cannot be discussed at this meeting pending a court case. What we can say is that trying to protect yourself from harm is a perfectly reasonable defence in the eyes of the law."

"What - stabbing someone in the arse is a reasonable response?" bawled the area's only remaining butcher, to snorts of laughter.

"What about keeping quiet for a minute and giving our invited guests a chance to speak!" shouted Frank.

Bill Howarth walked across the stage to a flip-chart which had the enigmatic slogan: "One In Four" scrawled across it.

Theatrically, the deputy director said: "One in four...one in four. That's the risk all of us run of having a mental illness at some time in our lives. All of you will have friends and relatives who suffer from depression, eating disorders, agoraphobia, schizophrenia...or are perhaps just off work with stress.

"Good old stress - we've all had that one. You might say it covers a multitude of ups and downs and family break-ups. But stress can lead to any one of these more serious conditions. And all of them might result in the need for professional help from a therapist or a psychologist – even a visit to a psychiatric hospital. But these quiet 'consultations' hardly ever show up on the sick note to work.

"What we all need to bear in mind is that mental ill health is all around us. Your next door neighbour; the woman you sit with in the canteen; even the boss in the office..."

Frank thought the deputy director must be a member of some amateur dramatic group the way he delivered his message. The audience fidgeted but listened. Then Winston was asked to get up and give his point of view. He explained how he'd been making coffee and none of the tenants had meant to hurt anybody – although they just got so much hassle all the time from complete strangers. "When I was locked up I got on with nearly everybody. As soon as they realised I was just like them nobody bothered me at all…" said Winston, half-wondering whether one of his Knock, Knock jokes would lighten the mood.

"You mean when you were in the hospital under Section," said Frank, smiling knowledgeably.

"No man, when I was in prison for that bit of bother…just a misunderstanding y'understand." Suddenly nobody did understand. The word 'prison' dropped like a beautifully gift-wrapped bomb into the laps of the mob at the back. The rumblings started immediately.

In an instant Bill Howarth stepped up beside Winston and shouted: "Hear him out…"

"Hear him out, let's bloody get him out," yelled a pensioner on the left .

"You never told us they was jailbirds as well as loonies, did you Mister deputy director?"

Other voices at the back began to chant: "Out, Out, Out…."

Concerned people at the front began to look round nervously and reach for their coats. Winston, getting more anxious by the second, called out: "But you're not listening!"

"Out, Out, Out...." chorused the men at the back, who'd been joined by a few women. Cans of lager were passed along the row.

Frank said lamely: "Can I remind everyone that this hall does not have a licence, you cannot drink alcohol in here."

But it was all too late and he knew it. Those prepared to listen were drowned out by the rabble who'd been on some sort of organised mission right from the start. No doubt pals of the three who'd been arrested.

A ghetto blaster was brought into the room and some of the men began jigging up and down. The night was theirs. And everyone in the two back rows knew there'd be a few free pints in the Queen's Head with Brian and Ian Beddows.

*****

By 9pm the Co-op hall was cleared. The councillors and social services' chief were the only ones left to push the chairs to the sides of the wall. Even though few dances were held on the perfectly sprung floor, the Co-op manager liked the place kept presentable to show prospective golden wedding couples.

At Peacehaven Mansions, Jane and Bella were settling down to watch a repeat of the Royle Family on television. Bella had finished her homework and Ray - newly discharged and sober as a judge - had presented them with delicious aubergine flowers in batter with a side order of his special chop suey…followed by rhubarb crumble and custard.

"Mesdames, you both know this is not my usual five star cuisine. However, I do believe theese is a selection of your personal favourites," joked Ray, adopting a terrible French accent. His cracked ribs were healing well. He was such a different character without a drink inside him.

After the television programme was finished he'd been teasing Jane about how chop suey wasn't remotely oriental. At some stage he'd gone back to his place for an old recipe book to prove his point. Then he'd become engrossed in a football game on ITV1 and fallen asleep in his armchair. After the heavy meal Bella and Jane both felt tired. When Ray didn't come back they decided to have an early night.

By 10pm Bella was asleep in the bedroom. In the lounge the Marlon Brando season was still going strong and Jane was drooping in front of On The Waterfront. She'd taken to recording her usual afternoon cinema choices because Bella nearly always arrived home in the middle of something good, then wanted to know what had happened earlier.

"Home," funny to think of this squalid little one-room flat as home, Jane realised. She'd never really thought of it in quite those terms until now. Perhaps having a child around made if feel more like a permanent place. Maybe she should think about getting some redecorating done.

As she stood at the front door enjoying what she promised herself would be the last cigarette of the night, Jane failed to notice the shadowy figure crouched behind a patch of high nettles.

Chapter 26

It was cold in the garden and Ken Cracknell was glad of the hip flask in the pocket of his old herringbone overcoat. Both the flask and the coat had been gifts from the daughter of the late Colonel Smythe when she'd been clearing out Peacehaven Mansions.

It was nearly 50 years since the retired army toff had judged Ken's allotment at the Cranmere and district annual show. That was in the days when the place had an annual show. After the prize-giving the colonel had offered Ken the chance to get out of the pits forever and enter a kind of horticultural heaven, growing flowers, vegetables and soft fruit in the grounds of this great old house.

After the fight in the garden Ken had kept his distance from the Queen's Head crowd, preferring to drink at home. He knew the garden well enough to slip away from the law. It used to be completely surrounded by a brick wall. Now there were two or three loose panels in the flimsy bit of fencing separating a wide strip at the back sold off for 'starter homes'. At his age Ken didn't want to get involved in any court proceedings. But in his head he couldn't escape the feeling he had let the Beddows   brothers down. Perhaps the whole neighbourhood.

Ken remembered Peacehaven Mansions when people who were worth something lived there. The grounds had been the house's great glory with herbaceous borders full of lupins, delphiniums and climbing roses. In autumn his dahlias had been spectacular and in the springtime the drifts of crocus, daffodils, then tulips, were better than any he'd seen at the newsagents in glossy gardening magazines.

There'd been no wheelie bins overflowing with rubbish waiting for collection at the front door. This hadn't been a place for nutters, jailbirds, coloured people and scruffy drunks stumbling up and down the driveway.

Ken revisited his old garden quite often at night. Nobody heard him, not with that racket going in the upstairs rooms most times. Some of the rambling roses survived and still gave off powerful scents. Once he took a pair of secateurs and clipped off the dead wood. His determination to get rid of the loonies had wavered only once. When he spotted a patch of newly-dug earth round the back where one of the women seemed to be trying to grow something.

Ken didn't recognise the leaf but pinched a bit off and took it home to examine. None of his gardening manuals identified the plant. But someone in the pub did and Ken nearly choked on his pint.

For once, it was quiet out here. No noise from the rooms upstairs, just a whiff of perfume coming from an old rose named in honour of the Queen Mother. Ken couldn't get to the main entrance without the risk of being noticed, but the flats on the side had their own front doors. One stood open for a while before being closed, and a bolt drawn across. It had to be the drunk's place. The former miner waited a long time after hearing the bolt, then a light in the bedroom being switched on, then off again. Finally, he crept forward.

Under his breath Ken muttered: "Good riddance, good riddance to the lot of you."

Fumbling for a few seconds, he unscrewed a green weedkiller bottle then, with all his joints aching, he bent almost double to quietly push open the small cat door and pour the contents onto the floor. There was no sound, the fluid must have been absorbed into a carpet. Next, Ken struck a match and threw that through the gap. He saw the flare and felt the heat as he straightened up and began backing away.

*****

Everyone smoked in the old black and white films, especially the thrilling war-time epics and gangster movies. On The Waterfront was the 1950s film that made the young Marlon Brandon a star. Jane loved him standing up for the dock workers' rights in downtown New York. It felt almost is if the fog from the river was drifting in off the screen as she began to doze, thinking how cosy the room had become.

I'm too ill to give up smoking, she sighed, making a mental note to empty all the ashtrays before

Bella come in the next morning. I bet she's got that cat in the bedroom again, she thought, snuggling down on the sofa, her right arm waving the remote control vaguely in the direction of the television.

It wasn't until some time later, when the bathroom window smashed in, that Jane woke up again, choking. The room was full of black smoke, there was a loud buzzing noise and she could hear Bella coughing and screaming from somewhere a long way away.

"Bella! Bella! Where are you?" Jane yelled.

But her voice didn't come out as a yell, more of a gasp as smoke caught her lungs and she found herself fighting for breath. Which was the way out....for Christ's sake which was the way out! Gulping and choking, Jane fought to clear her mind. She staggered blindly forward and banged into something solid. The table, it had to be the table...so if she went left...no right...her heart banged out of all control in her chest...right, right...she began to feel whoosy. If only that alarm would stop she could concentrate...

Another loud smash, closer this time, offered a glimmer of light. A figure staggered into the room...its face was masked and it threatened her with a stick.

"Oh God, not them again," gasped Jane as the man shot out an arm and grabbed her.

Through the fog she could see his eyes were contorted with fury, the face disguised with a blue rag showed some sort of cartoon illustration

of…What? Lisa Simpson!   Who were these animals?   The man began pulling her.
"No…no…." Jane bit and fought like she was possessed. Then he whacked her with the stick, and everything went dark.

*****

"Aunty Jane, Aunty Jane… speak to me, please wake up."
Jane was having a nightmare that involved her being back in the ECT room at the hospital. Drowsily she opened her eyes and realised she was in the open air and soaking wet. A man in a helmet was pressing something to her face. What? Oh, an oxygen mask.
The man pulled up the visor to his helmet and smiled. Even in the dark she could see one of his front teeth was missing. The fireman stared at her intently, holding her hand. No, he was checking her pulse. And Bella, lovely Bella, was there wide-eyed and clutching something that was wriggling in her arms….oh yes, the cat.
As soon as she saw Jane open her eyes Bella starting laughing with relief.
"They gave Mr C a quick burst of oxygen as well," she grinned.
Wendy was next: "Oh Jane what a relief! What a relief! But Jane, how many times have I asked you tenants not to smoke in bed?"
"Why am I so wet?" murmured Jane.

"'Cos you're sittin' on the wet grass love," said the gap-toothed fireman.

"Come on now, up you get, easy now, just go steady for a bit. You've had a lucky escape. You all have."

"It was Roger," gabbled Bella incomprehensibly. "It was Roger who saved us all.   He's back from France and was just walking up the path when he saw the smoke pouring out of my window and he had to smash the glass because the front door was a mass of flames.

"He climbed in and grabbed me and pushed me through the broken glass. I think Ray got me and Mr C leaped right out. Anyway, then I ran to Wendy and she dialled 999 and, and I saw Roger tie my pyjama jacket round his face and he turned back to find you. He's a hero."

"He was certainly in the right place at the right time," said the fireman. We'll be recommending him for an award – he deserves one going in with that walking stick and getting you both out of that window. Nobody could have got out of the front door."

*****

From the back of the garden Ken Cracknell had seen everything. At first he'd been furious when he saw the late-night visitor shouting and smashing the window. But when he heard the screaming, and realised there was a kiddie trapped inside, he'd felt ashamed. He'd gone too far and he knew it.

The flames were already licking up the side of the house. Why was everyone being so slow to hear the noise of that smoke alarm? Warily, Ken had crept up to the window and was in time to reach up and grasp the coughing and spluttering child being dangled over the ledge. Finally there were shouts and feet clanging on the fire escape above. A door opened in one of the other flats. Ken put the sobbing kiddie down and made his way back up the garden, slipping out through the loose fencing panel at the end.

*****

The night seemed to go on forever. Wendy, half relieved, half full of reproach, fussed over Roger as if he was her long-lost brother.

"I suppose she doesn't get out much," Jane muttered darkly to Bella, who wondered whether she ought to be doing more to safeguard her mum's romantic interests.

The rescue had taken more out of Roger than he cared to admit.

He told Jane: "I knew it was late to be calling but there was this great blues band playing in the city centre and I know you never go to bed early. I only stayed for their first set. Lucky I didn't stay for the second half."

Leaning more heavily on his stick, Roger was grateful to collapse onto a settee in Wendy's flat where he coughed for most of the night. The caretaker's place stank of the awful burning smell from next door but seemed otherwise unaffected. Ray and Renee's places were also okay although George's flat, directly above Jane's, had its windows blown out with the heat. George said he could cope and promised not to play any music. Jane and Bella took temporary refuge with Ray.

Chapter 27

At 8am the next day a reporter and photographer from the Evening Echo knocked on Ray's door. The reporter had already made the routine 7am calls to the police, fire and ambulance services to check on anything happening overnight. This dramatic rescue of a woman and child sounded like tonight's front page to him.

Their editor recognised the address and advised the pair to try to avoid the caretaker. She'd been the one who'd made all that fuss about the knife attack last week. What sort of place was this?

It was easy to spot which was the caretaker's flat. Scorched wheelie bins everywhere and just one door with a singed flowering basket – dead giveaway. The fire brigade had already supplied most of the details. All they really needed was a quick interview and a picture of the people plucked from the flames thanking the have-a-go-hero with the walking stick. But to make that night's edition they needed to get a move on. The evening paper had moved its print deadline to the stupidly early 10.30am.

Despite knocking and ringing most of the bells, sleepy Bella was the only resident of Peacehaven Mansions who actually opened a door. The reporter knew he couldn't interview the child without an adult so he urged her to get her mother – sorry, Aunty, was it? - out of bed.

Bella disappeared, then came back, saying it was impossible. Next the reporter asked whether she knew the man who'd saved her?

"He must be your hero, I guess."
Bella beamed and nodded. Obediently, she led
them to Wendy's flat and reached up to ring the
bell. Damn, it was the one with the flowers.
Fortunately, the door was answered by Roger,
leaning on his stick and scratching his head. The
cameraman took his chance and flashed off a few
pictures.
Half-confused about who these people were,
Roger just told them he'd only done what anyone
else would have done in the circumstances and
would prefer not to talk about it.
"It was nothing," said Roger, trying to pull Bella
inside and close the door. "Yes, I'm a
musician…how old am I? I don't know, about
39…playing with Who What in the city centre -
come and see us sometime. No really, I don't want
a fuss…."
"Pity we can't use a picture of the child," said the
photographer, as the pair hurried back to the
office.
"He'll do – local rock musician saves two," said the
reporter. "And didn't the kid say he was her hero.
Good enough for me."

*****

It was nearly 10am before the station officer from
Green Watch arrived and asked them all to cram
into Wendy's flat.
"I'm afraid this wasn't an accidental fire, as we first
thought," explained the fire chief.

Knock Knock, Who's There?

Some form of accelerant, almost certainly petrol, was poured directly onto the carpet, then set on fire. You're all very fortunate indeed.

The firefighter took a deep breath, then added: "There is no doubt in my mind we'd be looking at some fatalities if Mr Bailey here hadn't come along when he did. I take my hat off to you, sir."

"He's my Mum's boyfriend," said Bella, giving a meaningful glance in Wendy's direction.

"And that's this lady here, is it?" said the officer, looking at Jane, who had just managed to light up. Her hands felt weak and useless.

"No," said practically everybody in the room, each voice echoing the other and going up a scale with Jane's highest of all.

The fire chief shrugged.

"I'm sure you all have your own arrangements," he said, studying the faces of Jane, Ray, George, Amanda, Winston, Wendy, Roger and Bella.

"You can expect a visit from the police later this morning. This was a deliberate arson attack and we need to catch the person, or persons, responsible as soon as possible. All I can tell you is that whoever did this must be totally insane!"

The fire chief's words fell into a silent pool, as the tenants of Peacehaven Mansions turned solemnly to study each other.

Realising he'd made what could be an embarrassing social gaffe, or at least a politically incorrect one, the fireman hurried on to explain that detectives would be visiting the house shortly to start their enquiries. Hesitantly, he added: "I understand most of you, ahem, don't have jobs and so will be available when the police arrive."

"No, I'm afraid we won't," said Roger, struggling up from the settee and putting his smoke-blackened walking stick cautiously on the floor. "If somebody has tried to set this house on fire I want to take get this child out right away. She can come back with me to her mother's house – you too Jane, you need to get away from here."

"No, I don't," said Jane.

"Of course, you do. Don't you understand, somebody tried to kill you all?" How dense was this woman! Suddenly Roger had a glimpse of Sandy's frustrations with Jane and began to get angry.

Jane knew she was being irrational. She knew she probably owed her life to her sister's bloke but now here he was, automatically taking patronising control over her affairs. And her niece.

"Bella is perfectly capable of deciding what she wants to do," declared Jane. "But I'm staying right here to get to the bottom of this. My friends are here and Ray, or Renee, will put me up, won't you?

Both nodded dumbly.

"You must be out of your cotton-pickin' mind!" said Roger. "This isn't fantasy island any more Jane this is real ruddy life, your flat is uninhabitable and there are people out there who want to hurt you. And Bella. Think about Bella!"

"Please Aunty Jane, please come with us to Mum's house," pleaded Bella. "I'm scared."

Knock Knock, Who's There?

The child was tear-stained and worn out. Jane hated to see her like this but she realised Peacehaven Mansions was now her home. It was no use her trying to hide in leafy suburbia with Sandy. These were her friends, she had to stay and find out who hated her so much they wanted to kill her. Perhaps kill everyone in the house, including an innocent child. It had to be those Beddows brothers. But why?

"I'm staying for the moment," repeated Jane, stroking Bella's hair. "But you go with Roger and get some rest. I'll try and come and see you later."

The sub officer from Green Watch interrupted.

"I'd be grateful if you'd all just hang on a little while and give your statements to the police. This is arson and…perhaps attempted murder. We have to find out who did this terrible thing."

"We already know who did it!" said Jane sourly.

"All the more reason to tell the police about your suspicions," pointed out the fireman.

Wendy said: "Would anybody like a coffee?"

"No thanks," said Roger. "I've already told you all I know - there's nothing more I can add. Get your stuff Bella."

Chapter 28

The police promised to investigate Jane's theories about the arson attack but were dubious about any arrests.

"Doesn't sound like the Beddows brothers' style to me," said a world-weary detective from CID. They're not all that bright but not completely stupid."

"Not when they're already on bail for assault," added his partner.

The policemen weren't happy about Roger and Bella leaving what they described as the 'crime scene', but took Sandy's address and agreed to catch up with them later. The interview took place in Ray's flat. After they left Jane, who was having trouble covering herself with Ray's size zero dressing gown, started to cry.

"I've got used to having Bella around," she snuffled. "Now she'll never want to stay here again."

"Course she will, as soon as they catch these filthy creeps," said Ray. "Anyway, you should have gone with them. It's not right a young girl staying with a man who isn't her father or any other relative."

"Sandy trusts him."

"Jane, time to wake up. Stop worrying about yourself and start worrying about that child."

A sober Ray was a bit much to take when it was still only 11.30am. He was obviously still shaken by what had happened.

Knock Knock, Who's There?

"Even if last night wasn't down to the Beddows brothers, they've won. I'm drinking at home from now on. I'm not going anywhere near them or their precious Queen's Head – neither are you if you've got any sense. And before you start making random accusations, don't forget the police could still have you for wounding."

"But I can't stand Roger!" snapped Jane.

"And I can't stand my flat being full of smoke," Ray shouted back. "So go on, do the right thing. And if I manage to stay off the booze tonight I'll get the bus up there tomorrow. Bella needs you."

*****

The taxi didn't take long. It always surprised Jane how near she lived to her "oh-so-successful" sister's side of the city. A little oasis of perfect front lawns and manicured hedges. It always seemed like a million miles away from Jane's own world of illiterate graffiti and heavily-fortified corner shops. Sandy's house backed on to the edge of a cricket field. Local kids abandoned their mountain bikes in the shrubbery while they went inside to spend hours gathered round each other's latest computer games. The bikes would have been nicked in the first five minutes of being left on any street in Cranmere.

At least there everyone minded their own business. Whenever Jane ventured into this well-groomed wealth-belt it always seemed that everyone had time to stop and stare, question and pry into every crevice of her life.

"Oh, you're Sandy's sister aren't you? they'd say. "How is she?" Then there'd be a pause before the inevitable: "And how are you?"

Despite the kids leaving their expensive bikes all over the place, nearly every tree had a notice proclaiming: "This Is A Neighbourhood Watch Area."

On her last visit Jane had taken against the manager of the local café-bar who'd looked down his nose and asked her, icily, if she would put out her cigarette even when she was only sitting outside next to a patio heater!

Of course, Sandy said she loved the community spirit. She felt safer with all that Neighbourhood Watch stuff and fewer traffic fumes. Not that she'd felt all that happy about everyone knowing whenever Roger stayed the night…oh no…recalled Jane with a smirk. The curtain twitchers had been working overtime since he'd arrived on the scene. Roger certainly gave them something else to gossip about. At least it took some of the pressure off her with their endless questions.

The latest news was that Sandy would be out of hospital any day now.

"But can I stick it out until she gets here?" Jane muttered to herself before telling the taxi driver to pull up outside the house with the alpine-style shutters on the windows. Sandy always had loved Heidi books.

Knock Knock, Who's There?

Inside the house Bella heard the taxi pulling up and came running down the front path to greet her aunt.

"I knew you'd come Aunty Jane. Come in, come in, you can have that bedroom next to mine at the back. What did the police say? Are they after me and Roger? Will we have to give our statements…"

"Jane, just in time for a beer," said Roger, looking far too cosy as he appeared at the front door with a can in one hand and his stick in the other.

Jane paid off the taxi driver - £7 flaming 60p – he needn't even think about a tip. Then she squared her shoulders and marched up the path dragging her large, half-empty suitcase.

She told Bella: "I've only come for tonight, and maybe tomorrow, we'll see how it goes. Your Mum'll be back any minute."

"What about the police, Aunty Jane? What did you tell them? Have they caught anybody yet?"

"Caught anybody!" Jane could hardly keep the sarcasm out of her voice. "They can't usually catch a cold round our way. It's a bit different round here though," she added, nodding towards next door's tree with its "We are watching" friendly reminder notice.

*****

After Roger had cooked a reasonably tasty spaghetti bolognese, he told Jane: "I'm glad you've decided to stay because I really do need to go out tonight and find out about some work. My finances aren't what they were."

"Funny time to go looking for a job, in the middle of the night," said Jane.

"And when else do musicians work?" replied Roger, reaching for his coat and simultaneously shouting over his shoulder: "Remember, you promised only two or three fags in the house and the rest in the garden."

The door banged shut. All at once, Jane felt alone, and a little scared. Misunderstanding her expression, Bella whispered: "It's okay Aunty Jane, I won't tell if you have more than three cigarettes in the house – I'm used to it now. Roger's only worried Mum will make a fuss when she gets back. But she'll understand, I know she will."

From her suitcase Jane produced a video of Brief Encounter. Bella had developed quite a taste for black and white films and a few lessons in sexual restraint might be quite educational. Unfortunately, Sandy only had a DVD player so they agreed to watch Jungle Book instead. They were just settling down when there was loud knock on the door. After gripping each other in a quick panic, Bella crept to the front window and announced: "It's the police."

A uniformed policeman, aged about 18, stood on the doorstep. He was accompanied by an older woman, in plain clothes. Or else she was his mother, thought Jane. In which case she ought to give him some advice about his acne.

Knock Knock, Who's There?

"Mrs Bradstock," said the young policeman. "We're here about the fire at Peacehaven Mansions."

"We're from Cranmere and district police station," added his mum.

"It's Miss Wilson," replied Jane, stiffly. "And I've already given a statement this morning."

"Ah, it was a Miss Bradstock and Mr Roger Bailey, we particularly wanted to see," said the young officer. "We feel they may have information that might prove important to our enquiries."

"I'm afraid Mr Bailey's out," said Jane. "But he already gave a statement   to the fireman who came round last night. Roger didn't see anything or anyone, he just saw the smoke pouring out of Bella – my niece's window – the window in my flat that is, and smashed the glass."

"Could we come in a moment?" asked the policewoman, in a voice that made it clear this wasn't a request.

Jane opened the door wider to reveal Bella, listening in the hall.

"This is Bella Bradstock, my niece, she's had a terrible shock and will be going to bed soon," said Jane, trying to match the other woman's assertiveness.

"But I haven't given my statement yet," said Bella, caught up in the excitement of being involved in yet another police investigation. The first time they'd hardly taken any notice of her but now she was one of the main witnesses.

"Would you like some tea?" she asked, knowing it was what her mother would say and pretending not to notice her aunt's raised eyebrows.

"That would be very nice," said the policewoman, introducing herself as Detective Inspector Maria Perkins.

"Well, I'd better make it then, hadn't I?" said Jane looking meaningfully at Bella, "while you start giving your statement."

"Miss Wilson I'd rather you remained in the room while we interview a minor," said Det. Insp. Perkins crisply.

As it happened Bella's information took the arson investigation no further at all. She remembered the window smashing, she remembered the smoke and she remembered a man she later realised was Roger slapping her awake.

"I hit him back at first," she confessed. "Of course, I didn't know it was Roger trying to save me – he's my Mum's boyfriend. Well, fiancé, he isn't a boy."

It seemed Roger had shouted for all he was worth then smashed the glass and climbed in through Jane's bedroom window. He'd dragged Bella out of bed, thrown a towel over the jagged panes of glass then handed her back through the window.

"I think maybe he handed me to Ray because it was somebody who smelt a lot of beer," explained Bella. "Then he ripped my pyjama top off and tied it round his head and I saw him open the bedroom door. Even in the dark I could see there was loads of smoke pouring out of the hallway...Roger kept shouting 'Jane, Jane'...but Aunty Jane isn't good at waking up…." Bella glanced anxiously at her aunt, worried she'd betrayed a secret.

"Then Roger just ran right through all that smoke and pulled Aunty Jane out. She was unconscious when he dragged her back to the window and pushed her out just as two firemen ran up the drive. We were both really lucky…"

Bella would have gone on but suddenly checked herself and became thoughtful.

"Somebody was trying to kill us, weren't they?" She turned to Jane and started to cry.

"Shhh, shush…they weren't trying to kill you lovely, what have you done to anybody? They're just sick people who need locking up far more than I ever did."

"You were locked up, madam?" said the young policeman. "Can I ask why?"

Jane glared at him. "For being a nutcase," she sighed, reaching for her cigarettes. "But not as big a nutcase as those swines who tried to burn the house down."

"But you have been down at the police station recently, I believe," put in Det Insp. Perkins, evenly. "There is a court case pending, I understand."

"That's right, and you'll find the same   thugs who attacked one of the other tenants in Peacehaven Mansions, just the other day, were also responsible for last night's little affair. These are extremely violent people."

"You're referring to the charges brought against Ian and Brian Beddows?" said the policewoman. "I'm afraid we've already spoken to them earlier this evening and both have pretty cast-iron alibis about where they were at the time of this fire."

"Don't tell me, in the Queen's Head," said Jane, finding it hard to strike a match.

"That's right."

"Oh I still think you'll find they're behind it. Even if they didn't personally pour the petrol onto my hall carpet. They hate us. All of us. They can't stand the notion of a half-way house for mental defectives being shoved in the middle of their already crime-ridden community."

"I think you'll find 'crime-ridden' is perhaps where we have the problem," said Det Insp Perkins. "You see there's been so much trouble in Cranmere lately that any number of people could be responsible for this sort of attack."

"But there are only a few with a track record for arson," added the young officer, before glancing nervously at his senior officer wondering if he'd revealed too much.

Ignoring him, she repeated: "When will Mr Bailey be back?"

"I should imagine not until after midnight," said Jane. "He's a musician – plays late at night in bars."

"Do you happen to know his current address?"

Jane shrugged but Bella, still tearful, said: "Mum's got his address in her book. But he's staying with us until she gets out of hospital. They had a car crash - in France."

"You don't seem to be having very much luck at the moment," observed Det Insp. Perkins. Jane was glad to see her tone softened, as she addressed the child.

"Suppose we don't," said Bella, copying Roger's address out on a piece of paper and handing it over.

"Right, well, I think that's it. Do tell Mr Bailey that we are very anxious to speak to him," said the policewoman, "perhaps he could give the office a ring in the morning?"

Again, Jane knew this wasn't really a question.

"We'll tell him," she promised. "Goodnight."

Chapter 29

Roger turned out to be "helping the police with their enquiries", when Sandy, leaning heavily on Mary, walked carefully up the garden path late the following day.

Bella was beside herself with joy as Sandy hugged and hugged her precious daughter, and wept.

Eventually, she turned to her sister. "I can't thank you enough for all you've done Jane. You've been a tower of strength. Mum always said you'd be fine looking after Bella – I thought it would be too much for you to cope with on top of your own troubles. But look at her – she's…she's…" Sandy, the professional spokeswoman, was lost for words. She began sobbing again.

Several neighbours arrived to welcome the invalid home and promised to call back with hot dinners and lemon meringue pie. It was more than an hour later, after they'd all drank tea and Jane had smoked five cigarettes, that Sandy asked her daughter and sister the question they'd both been dreading.

She and Mary had been consuming bowl after bowl of breakfast cereal. The one food they'd desperately missed.

"What can have happened to Roger?"

"He erm, I think he's working…he didn't know you were arriving tonight…did he?" said Jane.

"That's right, you thought you wouldn't be coming back until tomorrow Mum, remember?" put in Bella.

Knock Knock, Who's There?

Sandy looked puzzled. "He seems to have vanished off the face of the earth in the past 24 hours. Until now he's been really good at keeping me up to date on what's been happening but I was ringing and texting all last night and got nowhere. I bet the batteries are flat on his mobile again. Either that or he's not got round to topping up his credit. Typical Roger! I expect he'll roll up in the middle of the night."

Mary said: "You look dead beat Sandy, perhaps it's time we helped you up to bed."

"No, not yet Mum. I want to find out more about what's been going on."

"Ooh lots, you don't know about the fire," said Bella. "Only, only because Aunty Jane and Roger didn't want to worry you...."

"What fire? Where?" said Sandy and Mary in alarmed tandem.

"This wasn't the time Bella," said Jane, lighting up another cigarette before trying to explain.

"It happened a couple of days ago. We think it was those Beddows' brothers again, you know the ones who beat Ray up before? Oh no, sorry, you don't know about that either. But don't worry, the police are on to them. Anyway, the thing is, we think one of them poured petrol through the cat flap."

"What!" Sandy and Mary seemed to choke, simultaneously.

"But Roger was a hero, he broke in and saved me and Aunty Jane - he might be going to get a medal," gabbled Bella.

"And you weren't hurt?" said Sandy, looking dazed.

"Course not Mum, you can see we're both fine,"

"What about Roger – is that why he's not here," said Mary. "Was he hurt?"

"No, no, he's with the police...oh...." Bella trailed off.

"What!" This time Mary just had the edge on Sandy in a joint cry of alarm.

"Okay, look, we'd better tell you the whole story," said Jane. "There's been some misunderstanding - although Roger brought it all on himself. The police kept trying to interview him about the fire – they just wanted his eye-witness account of what he saw when he arrived. But you know how 'casual' he can be sometimes?"

"How do you mean?" Sandy looked lost.

"Come on Sandy, you know he never takes anything very seriously. He's always having a quiet laugh at me even though you've told him I'm not well. Anyway, he'd already told the firefighters what happened on the night of this...this arson attack. He thought they could just pass on all his information to the police – he didn't see why he should have to go over it all again. Kept ranting on and on about endless paperwork, useless bureaucracy, didn't one emergency service ever talk to the other? Don't ask me why he was making such a big deal about it, but he was.

"Anyway, the result is they caught him packing a bag at his flat and got suspicious...I mean you can see it from their point of view. They didn't know he was only packing a bag to come here – they just saw him as this man who wouldn't go in for questioning. Then, when they finally catch up with him in his own home, well…in their eyes it must have looked like he was, well…doing a bunk."

"But why would he do that?" asked Mary. Sandy said nothing. She swallowed hard and her face was very pale.

Jane said: "Listen Sandy, it will all be sorted out in no time. Let's face it, he's probably going to turn up here later tonight."

For the first time in years, Mary found herself actively agreeing with her older daughter's assessment of a situation.

"Jane's right Sandy, this can all be sorted out easily. In the meantime the flight has really taken it out of you – it's time you got into bed."

To her surprise, Sandy just nodded dumbly, struggled out of the chair and headed for the stairs.

"I'll come up with you," said Mary. "But if I come and lie down beside you, I'm not going to suddenly find Roger crawling into bed with us, am I?"

Jane and Bella grinned faintly at the image, but Sandy didn't seem to catch her mother's almost risqué joke.

*****

Next morning it was the shouting that roused Jane from her usual sleep of the dead. The nearly hysterical voice was her sister's and she was

obviously talking on the telephone to someone
who was being less then helpful.

"What do you mean you're going to keep him in
custody for another 24 hours! "What do you
suspect him of doing? My sister's told you he
saved the lives of her and my daughter from a
house fire – he'd hardly have bothered to do that if
he'd started the thing would he?

"Yes, I know I'm being abusive! Just let me talk to
someone in charge - there must be a duty
inspector around somewhere.

"Yes, yes, I understand it's Sunday but the whole
police station can't come to a halt just because it's
Sunday, can it? Don't criminals commit any
crimes on Sundays? You'll be telling me next
they're all in church!

"Yes…yes, I am being sarcastic – why are you
holding my fiancé for a crime he can't possibly
have committed?

"What! "Say that again.   This is preposterous!
You've made some terrible mistake…All right, I'll
ring my solicitor – she'll come down I'm sure. Even
though it is Sunday…"

Sandy slammed the phone down as Jane knocked
on her bedroom door then rushed right in. She'd
never seen her sister looking so ill. Her face was
flushed and there were dark circles under her
eyes.

"They….they say they're questioning Roger about
another matter, nothing to do with the fire."

"What!"

"They're holding him in connection with something
else. They won't tell me what it is…"

Knock Knock, Who's There?

Sandy had begun shivering and weeping when the telephone rang again. The call was from France – the English-speaking doctor who had been so good to her was ringing to find out how she was. Stammering, Sandy explained she'd just had a bit of a shock and would ring back. Jane didn't know what to do except hold her. The two sisters clung to one another, not speaking, until Bella breezed in, half an hour later.

"Mum! What's the matter?"

"Bella, do us a favour and go and make a pot of tea will you?" whispered Jane hoarsely. "Your Mum'll be okay in a little while. Oh, and can you bring up my cigarettes and the address book? We need to get some legal advice."

Chapter 30

God, God, God....Roger felt like banging his head repeatedly on the wall of his flat. He had to go, but this time he really wanted to stay. Everything was different. He could have made it with Sandy. She was smart, she'd already had some ideas about promoting a national tour even though she knew bugger all about music. This woman could have sorted him out – given him space. And the kid was great - imaginative little player, loads of promise.

"Why do I always screw up?"

Slowly, it dawned on Roger that he really was banging his head on the wall. There would be no way back, and he knew it. He'd already packed a bag and looked up train timetables when he decided to plug in his guitar, connect the amp and start strumming.

Two of the tabloids had picked up the story about the fire from the Evening Echo. Just a column and a headshot: "Rock Musician Saves Two Lives." Hell, he wasn't even famous. It had to be a slow news day. But Jenny, or one of her friends, would spot it. The police would start asking more questions.

In the past all that ever mattered to him had been the music, making it, listening to it. Now he wanted more. Perhaps it was middle age creeping in. This time he'd really wanted Sandy. Maybe he could have even helped with that crazy sister of hers.

Knock Knock, Who's There?

Melancholy poured from Roger into the music. He decided he'd write Sandy a song. Perhaps that's all he could do for her now. He thought about their holiday in France, before the accident, about the colour of her eyes in the sunshine, his fingers reaching and finding chord combinations he hadn't used for years. And for once, the lyrics just flowed. Sandy's song, Turquoise, took just two hours to compose. When it was finished Roger knew it was one of the best pieces he'd written since the surprise chart-topper he'd done for The Warriors at the end of the 1980s. The royalties for that had seen him over a lot of rough patches during the artistically purer decade that followed.

Turquoise was easy on the ear. Perhaps now was the time to go in for a little commercial prostitution. He was certainly going to need the money.

Roger rang his London agent, Ben Zanda, and pressed the hands-free button so he could play the tune over the phone. For once Ben was immediately enthusiastic. He turned on his headphone recorder and asked Roger to play the song through twice more.

"If I wasn't Jewish I'd say you might just have saved my bacon," said Ben.

"What do you mean?"

"I've signed this new young band but they've been a nightmare getting together their first album. It should have been finished last month but they still need another couple of numbers. And I can't hear a single on any of the stuff they've laid down so far. This just might be the one. Look, I'll play this tape to them tonight – can you be in London tomorrow?"

Roger agreed to transcribe the notes for Turquoise onto his computer software and email the score to Ben along with a few other songs he'd been working on. They'd fixed a time to meet up before Roger confessed: "There's an outside chance I might not be able to make it. I seem to have a bit of unfinished business with the boys in blue to take care off."

"I didn't think you went in for any of those mind-altering substances," said Ben.

"You know I bloody don't," said Roger. "It's just the cops want to do some routine interview with me and that might lead on to them asking about other things. I saved a child from a fire. Some of the tabloids have picked up a picture of me. It's only a headshot but after all these years, Jenny in Lancashire seems to want to track me down."

"Tell me about it. Last summer I had private detectives sniffing around here asking about your whereabouts. Naturally I told them I didn't know where you were. Which was easy – because I didn't."

"That means the police are bound to have me on their missing person computers," groaned Roger. "Hell, it's not as if I've got any cash."

Ben, who had been Roger's agent for more than a decade, said:

"Correct me if I'm on the edge of Alzheimer's, but this is Mrs Bailey number two we're talking about, isn't it?"

"No such luck. It's Mrs Bailey number one. We never actually got round to getting divorced.
"Tricky."
"Yeah. I had to quit the music exam board after Jenny tried to trace me through them. By now she'll have got hold of Elaine in Brighton and told her all about my little marital oversight. I could be going down for this."
At the other end of the phone Ben blew the air from his cheeks.
"Bigamy. I give up! Why the hell didn't you just live with these women like everybody else does these days? I suppose that'd be too easy for you – always the romantic. How many more are there? This won't be a class action will it?"
"What do you take me for? Anyway, publish my stuff under someone else's name. "
Ben said: "I suppose it goes without saying that both Mrs Baileys are well-heeled ladies? Ones whose fathers have a few bob in the bank – enough to pay for good lawyers?"
"Yep, I'm screwed."
"And what about your new fiancée?"
"That's the sad bit. I really, really want to stay with this one. It was her kid I rescued. But Sandy's very straight, honourable. When she finds out about my other 'ladies', there'll be no way back. And all I did was become a local hero."
"Ah stay where you are man," said Ben. "Time to stop running. If you've been a hero then they're not ten a penny. Bet the judge'll go easy on you in court."

Roger wasn't convinced until Ben added: "Look, screw the nom-de-plume – if we're going to market this new record a little notoriety won't do you any harm at all."

Despite this advice Roger was still in a quandary about whether he should go round to face Sandy with the truth or to catch the next London train and try to explain things from the safety of his mobile phone, 100 miles away. Then the police arrived and left him no choice. Roger hadn't reckoned on his favourite pupil helpfully supplying them with the address of his flat. It seemed his reluctance to get in touch had led to a few "routine checks" explained Inspector Perkins, who thought it might be "more convenient" if he accompanied her back to the station.

The packed suitcase needed some explaining. At least his guitar was still plugged in.

Chapter 31

Wearing baggy trousers and seriously huge hoop earrings, Jane caught the bus up to see Sandy and Bella. Her flat still wasn't really habitable but once the glass had been put back in the window and a new door installed, Jane insisted she didn't care about the lingering smell of burning.
"I'm still waiting for the: 'I told you so'," said Sandy, struggling to lift one of Roger's spare amplifiers. She was far too weak and set it down again as Bella mutely followed her around the house carrying two supermarket bags bulging with what looked like shirts and CDs. Both mother and daughter were glum.
"I've made a few mistakes in my time," said Jane, her hands shaking as she lit up. She seemed to be suffering from some sort of delayed reaction to the fire. For more than a quarter of a century the conviction she was dying gradually, as a result of heart disease, had always weighed down some part of her mind. Her heart was far too weak to carry on much longer. Not with all the fags she smoked. Because it was already too late to give up.
Dying was the compass by which Jane had set the course on most of her adult life. Even without medical proof, the firm belief that she was terminally ill had offered some kind of refuge from the pointlessness of living. When things were bad, the thought of death was a comfort. On good days the knowledge lay snoozing, at the back of her brain, only roused if the voices broke in.

Now the idea that her life, pathetic though it was, could simply be wrenched away from her by some random arsonist, was totally unsettling. And not least because whoever was responsible, could strike again.

Jane heard herself saying: "Roger wasn't all bad. I mean I always thought he was dodgy but that was because I guessed he was hiding something. As it happened he was. Two people."

"Don't rub it in," sighed Sandy. "I won't be such a gullible fool next time. Not that there's ever going to be a next time."

"You'll meet someone – someone more like Tom, a solicitor - more your type…"

Sandy burst into tears.

"Bella, go and put the kettle on will you," said Jane. Up until the last few days, it had been years since she'd put a comforting arm around her little sister.

"I'm always putting the kettle on, you both keep shutting me out," moaned Bella.

"Then I'll put the kettle on," said Mary, coming downstairs. "Now, have you got all his bits and pieces?" She was careful not to mention Roger's name.

Nobody did. But Bella didn't mind saying his name. Bella still clung to some thread of hope that Roger might one day be reconciled with her mum. All right he hadn't told them he was still married. Or still married, twice. But he had made her mum happy. And he had saved her life. And Aunty Jane's life. He was an artist. He couldn't be expected to remember everything.

Chapter 32

Detective Inspector Maria Perkins was considerably kinder when she made her next visit to Sandy's house. Bella had left, morosely, for school and Sandy was lingering over her morning coffee, thinking she really ought to put in an appearance at the office.

She knew she wasn't well enough to actually do any work, but she still had a neglected business to run. A few clients were getting worried. Several considered themselves personal friends and had already clogged up her home answer phone with 'Get Well Soon,' messages.

Sandy's instinct for spotting good staff had been one of the reasons she'd scored so highly in the business awards earlier in the year. She had a natural talent for recognising individual strengths, balancing her small workforce and, if necessary, paying over the odds to keep them. Their loyalty over the past few weeks had reaped far higher benefits than she could have ever foreseen. Essentially, they'd kept her company solvent.

Pity I don't seem to have the same instinct when it comes to choosing a suitable boyfriend, she told herself.

It was Monday morning and Det Insp Perkins had come to explain that her "fiancé" had already been released from custody. This wasn't news to Sandy. Roger had been telephoning and texting her all night. Despising her own cowardice, Sandy simply hadn't felt strong enough to speak to him right then.

It had been her own solicitor who'd revealed the shocking news that Roger was being held as a suspected bigamist. Of course, it could have been so much worse. But when Sandy found out Roger appeared to have overlooked the existence of not one, but two ex-wives, it was as if a puzzle clicked into place and she knew it was true.

He wasn't an evil man; he was highly talented. Just totally feckless and self-absorbed. Roger lived for the moment, both on stage and in real life. He had that wonderful ability of making those around him feel so alive. He'd brought Sandy back to life, emotionally, which was why it hurt so much now.

"Would you like some tea?" she asked Det Insp. Perkins.

"That's just what your very polite young daughter asked me the first time I called at this address," smiled the policewoman, who explained the main reason for her visit was to see whether Sandy would have another word with Bella about the night of the fire.

"You see, we now think Mr Bailey actually passed your daughter through the window and right into the arms of the arsonist. We assume this was a man but it could well be that only Bella knows what he actually looks like," said Det Insp Perkins.

"I'll have another word with her," agreed Sandy. "Though I honestly think if she remembered anything other than the smell of alcohol on this person's breath, she would have told me. You've definitely ruled out it being Ray, the man next door?"

"Absolutely, he was still in his flat when the rescue started."

A shiver ran down Sandy's spine. "Then whoever the arsonist is, he's still out there. Which means my sister, and all the other people in Peacehaven Mansions, remain at risk from this madman. I suppose I have to be grateful he hung around long enough to help Bella out."

"We're keeping a careful watch on the property," said DI Perkins before adding: "I must admit I've been impressed by the rather amazing sense of spirit among those people at the house. I know they all have their problems but they've really banded together to watch out for each other. I understand they also looked after your daughter when you were in hospital."

Sandy blinked back the tears. "Yes, Bella was well looked after. My sister and her neighbours all face quite significant mental health issues. But rather like the people in my office, they pooled their resources and helped each other. Helped me, and my daughter. I must find some way of rewarding them. Perhaps take them all out for a meal…although that might not be entirely appropriate for Ray. D'you know, despite appearances, he's a very well-qualified chef?"

"Do you plan to get back in touch with Mr Bailey?" asked DI Perkins, delicately.

"Yes, of course," said Sandy. "I just couldn't face him last night. It was the shock. I, I, feel such a fool…"

"He's got a lot of personal charm," conceded the senior officer, who had three children and a policeman husband she hardly saw because of conflicting shift patterns.

Unprofessionally, she couldn't resist adding: "I can understand why anybody might fall for Mr Bailey."

Sandy looked at her with gratitude. She noticed DI Perkins had well-cut hair and discreetly applied light grey eye-shadow. She was probably about the same age as Jane, who rarely bothered with make-up, only earrings.

"In the fire, Roger really did save my daughter, and my sister, didn't he?" asked Sandy, feeling like she was grasping at straws.

The policewoman nodded. "I understand the fire service have put his name forward for an award. Although I fear these impending charges may alter things."

Empathising with Sandy's utter desolation, the policewoman added: "Look, I probably shouldn't be saying this, but from one woman to another, it might comfort you to know that Mr Bailey did speak very fondly of you when we had him in for questioning. He's obviously been a bit of a philanderer who's finally come face-to-face with all the hurt he's caused. To his credit he showed a considerable amount of remorse in the interview room – kept going on endlessly about how much he's let you down."

"What will happen to him?" asked Sandy.

DI Perkins shook her head: "Possibly a short prison term, more likely a heavy fine and a period of probation or community service. Then he'll have to deal with maintenance claims from his ex-wife, if they're valid, and any subsequent claims from

the second Mrs Bailey, who was suing for divorce
without realising she'd never been legally married.
Messy. At least there don't appear to be any
children involved."
The policewoman got up to leave.
Sandy said: "I'll speak to Roger today. And I'll
speak to Bella when she gets back from school -
see if she can remember anything else."

Chapter 33

"Roger."

"Sandy, is that you? Oh it's so good to hear your voice. How are you? Listen I'm so sorry...you can't imagine how sorry I am. I know, I know I'm a bastard. But getting to know you was fantastic....and then, well then I fell for you and somehow I couldn't risk blowing it."

"The truth might have been nice," said Sandy, her hand shaking as she sat in her bedroom holding the phone. Strictly a spritzer drinker during her many work-related cocktail parties, she'd already knocked back three gin and tonics.

"The truth would have made you run a mile," said Roger. "I'd blocked Jenny and Elaine out – they were the past. You.You and Bella were going to be my future. The sort of future I always wanted."

"Always wanted?"

"Okay, not always wanted. Wanted now, because of where I am in life. I've grown up. I must be the classic case of arrested development. Music mattered. Nothing else was really serious."

"Not relationships at any rate," said Sandy.

"Not until now. Until the one I have...had...with you. I even let the guys go on tour so I could stay with you."

"Or was that just to keep one step ahead of the private detective one of your wives had on your trail?" said Sandy, surprising herself with her determined cynicism, while inwardly wanting to scream.

Knock Knock, Who's There?

"It wasn't like that. Sandy, you know it wasn't like that. We had something together, you and me."

"But I can never trust you again."

"Not even if we took it really slowly? If we started all over again…just saw one another some times…perhaps after I'm properly divorced?"

"I don't think so."

"At least listen to the song I've written telling you how I feel. It's called Turquoise, after the colour of your eyes. Ben, my agent has got a young band he represents to record it. They've already had one hit and are looking for a follow-up. And there's other stuff I worked on when I was strumming with Bella. The lyrics just need a bit of polishing but Ben says they're commercial. I could be making some serious money, at last."

"Haven't you forgotten all the fines and maintenance payments you've saddled yourself with? Listen Roger, I'm going to leave all your things at Jane's flat. I think that would be for the best. I can't face seeing you at the moment and Bella will only be upset if you come to the house. She's almost as hurt as I am."

Roger's voice wavered. He blew his nose loudly. He said: "Ever since I left school I've moved on to new towns and cities, new bands, new people. For the first time I want to stay right here, in this city. I want to be with you. If that can't happen then at least I want to be in the same place as you. You won't mind that, will you?"

Sandy sighed. "I don't know what I mind, or what I think – except let down. More than that. Betrayed by somebody I thought I was going to spend the rest of my life with…who, who even my daughter had started to care about…."

"Listen, whatever happens, tell Bella to keep practising," said Roger, his voice thick with emotion. "And Sandy, I'll burn my new song onto a disc and send it to you. It's going on general release soon but it's your song. Listen to the lyrics. Can I call you sometime?"

"I don't know," said Sandy, replacing the receiver.

Chapter 34

"I think it's best if you just take your stuff and push off mate," Ray said to Roger when he called at Peacehaven Mansions to collect the clothes, CDs and toiletries he'd left lying around at Sandy's house. It had been three weeks since he'd seen her.

Two extra-large supermarket bags stood in the hall. It was raining hard and Roger found himself blinking back the tears at the thought of Sandy packing all his stuff. One bag contained his leather trousers, a shirt she'd bought him and a pair of trainers.

At the bottom was a wedge of heavily crossed-out and overwritten sheet music. A casual flick revealed some of the compositions were not his but Bella's. Sandy didn't recognise the difference. As he began fumbling, trying to extract the child's work, Ray told him he'd better come in out of the rain.

"I'll miss them both," said Roger, wondering where Jane was.

Ray, who hadn't had a drink for two days, said: "Yeah well, I'm not saying anything against you. We can't all be perfect and you saved two people's lives here. That's something you can be proud of."

"Have the police got any further in finding the guy in the big overcoat – the one I handed Bella to?"

Jane appeared from the bedroom. She had a cigarette in one hand and was brushing flecks of ash from her knee with the other. A disgruntled

Mr C stalked, stiff-legged, behind her, his tail swishing angrily. The three of them heard a small slap as he left through his recently replaced cat flap.

"No, they haven't found the man in the overcoat," said Jane. "And those Beddows brothers apparently don't own a full-length coat between them. So it looks like they're off the hook, unless you can remember anything more. I don't know why you ever thought it was Ray on the other side of the window."

Exasperated Roger said: "I didn't notice who the hell it was on the other side of the window – I only knew it was dark and that you must still be trapped in the other room. It was Bella who thought it was Ray because, because…"

Ray finished the sentence. "I know, because the fella smelt of booze. Well, there's a lot of us drinkers out there. But I'm beginning to think I've seen the bloke they want to question in the pub, except that he seems way too doddery to do anything like this. He always wears one of those heavy zig-zag patterned coats and not many people do these days. I've caught him glaring at me a few times before I've got too pissed to care."

"In that case those Beddows know who he is," said Jane.

"And d'ya think they'll tell?" said Ray, raising his eyebrow in a way Jane usually found funny. This time there was nothing to laugh about.

Instead she turned to Roger: "Listen, don't think I'm not grateful to you for saving my life, and Bella's. It's just that at the same time you seem to

have robbed my sister of some of hers. And to be honest, her life was worth a lot more than mine."
Roger had picked up the first bag when Jane added: "Sandy said something about not sending your electric toothbrush. Bit petty of her if you ask me. Still, I'm not sure she'll ever get over you; and Bella's as gloomy as can be. How could you be so cruel? Didn't you realise that Sandy had already lost her husband and brought up that child single-handed; then she'd started her own business...even tried her best to look after me. And now this. She doesn't deserve it!"
Somewhere in the middle of Jane's rant, a light bulb of hope flashed on in Roger's head.
Sandy hadn't sent his electric toothbrush. The one she'd insisted on buying after noticing his old one had lost most of its bristles. Roger had tried to tell her he really didn't need anything so special.
She'd laughed and said he was special. Now was she sending him a message? Did it mean that one day - one day soon - he just might be forgiven?
In a daze, Roger handed over Bella's music. "Encourage her to keep trying to compose her own material. She's a clever kid," he said.
All three of them stood awkwardly in the hall: Ray wondering whether he should offer to shake Roger's hand; Jane desperately wanting this life-saving stranger to turn into the sort of man her sister could marry; and Roger wondering, just wondering, if he'd read the signs right.
The cat flap slapped again and Mr C strolled back in with a slug caught on the back claw of his left

leg. Despite the animal's best endeavours, he was having trouble shaking it off.

"I see you're still having a problem with other slimy invaders?" said Roger, grimacing at his own feeble joke. He put his hands up: "Don't worry, I'm going, I'm going."

From the door Jane watched Roger reach the end of the drive, then turn to walk down the main road. Some maudlin' new release, Turquoise, was being played on the radio upstairs as Jane, feeling close to tears, tilted back her head and bellowed:

"George, I've got a job for you."

*****

After the disposal job, Jane tried to relax. Compared to Brian and Ian Beddows, the slugs were really no problem at all. Next month the brothers were due up in court for their assault on Ray. What were the chances they'd appear at the same time as bigamist Roger? Oh no, she forgot, his case was back in Brighton, where the second Mrs Bailey lived.

The police had already warned that some plea bargaining had gone on and so while Jane had been let off with a caution, the charges against the two brothers and Brett Ansley had been reduced. These were no longer assault with intent to cause grievous bodily harm, but the less serious, assault with intent to cause actual bodily harm.

Knock Knock, Who's There?

They'd still had the gall to plead not guilty. Unless any of them had a long record of previous offences, any penalty imposed by the city magistrates was unlikely to get them off the streets. At least not for long.

Thinking about the attack, Jane felt so angry on Ray's behalf – and on behalf of all the tenants of Peacehaven Mansions – that she ignored the familiar palpitations in her chest.

Instead she got up and said to Ray: "Fancy some tea and toast?"

Of course, she was out of butter. But Ray had some. As he dodged back through the showers to his flat, Ray failed to notice the pensioner in the herringbone overcoat who stood on the edge of the drive and spat in the shrubbery. Ken Cracknell would never accept the tragic fate of this fine house that had not only provided him with a livelihood outside the pit but an outlet for all his creative aspirations. He was done with the place now. Let the loonies have it.

Only Renee and George, in their upstairs flats were looking down onto the rain-soaked road. George had switched off some sad dirge on the radio then cranked up the volume on his hi-fi for some full-blast Status Quo.

Before being summoned to his slug removal job, George had been sorry to see Roger heading off, his carrier bags bulging with the sort of classic CDs he would have loved to copy. Renee had always taken her cue from Jane when it came to Roger. She decided she'd never really liked him.

Nor did she like the look of this old bloke outside, glaring up at the building. No doubt another one muttering to himself about it being Fruitcake Towers. Renee knew she'd seen him before so he must live locally. She pulled the curtains. People were always watching the house.

Printed in the United Kingdom
by Lightning Source UK Ltd.
127716UK00001BA/97-108/P